OPCS Surveys of Psychiatric
Morbidity in Great Britain

Report 7

Psychiatric morbidity among homeless people

Baljit Gill

Howard Meltzer

Kerstin Hinds

Mark Petticrew

London: HMSO

Notice

On 1 April 1996 the Office of Population Censuses and Surveys and the Central Statistical Office merged to form the Office for National Statistics. The logo of the new Office appears on the front cover of this report but the report series name - 'OPCS Surveys of Psychiatric Morbidity in Great Britain' - remains unchanged, to preserve the continuity of the 8-report series. Reference to OPCS inside the report are also unchanged since it was already in production at the time of the merger.

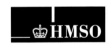

Published by HMSO and available from:

HMSO Publications Centre
(Mail, fax and telephone orders only)
PO Box 276, London SW8 5DT
Telephone orders 0171 873 9090
General enquiries 0171 873 0011
(queuing system in operation for both numbers)
Fax orders 0171 873 8200

HMSO Bookshops
49 High Holborn, London WC1V 6HB
(counter service only)
0171 873 0011 Fax 0171 831 1326
68–69 Bull Street, Birmingham B4 6AD
0121 236 9696   Fax 0121 236 9699
33 Wine Street, Bristol BS1 2BQ
0117 9264306 Fax 0117 9294515
9–21 Princess Street, Manchester M60 8AS
0161 834 7201 Fax 0161 833 0634
16 Arthur Street, Belfast BT1 4GD
01232 238451 Fax 01232 235401
71 Lothian Road, Edinburgh EH3 9AZ
0131 228 4181 Fax 0131 229 2734
The HMSO Oriel Bookshop
The Friary, Cardiff CF1 4AA
01222 395548 Fax 01222 384347

HMSO's Accredited Agents
(see Yellow Pages)

and through good booksellers

Authors' acknowledgements

We would like to thank everybody who contributed to the survey and the production of this report. Organisations concerned with the welfare of homeless people as well as administrators and care workers in the hostels, daycentres and nightshelters were of great assistance to the OPCS interviewers not only in organising contact with respondents but helping as proxy informants when subjects could not manage an interview.

We were supported by our specialist colleagues in OPCS who carried out the sampling, field-work, coding and editing stages.

The project was steered by a group comprising the following, to whom thanks are due for assistance and specialist advice at various stages of the survey:

Department of Health:
Dr Rachel Jenkins (chair)
Dr Terry Brugha
Ms Antonia Roberts
Mr Alan Madge

Psychiatric epidemiologists:
Professor Paul Bebbington
Professor Glyn Lewis
Dr Mike Farrell
Dr Jacquie de Alarcon

Office of Population Censuses and Surveys:
Ms Jil Matheson
Dr Howard Meltzer
Ms Baljit Gill
Ms Kerstin Hinds
Dr Mark Petticrew

Most importantly, we would like to thank all the participants in the survey for their co-operation.

Contents

List of tables

List of figures

Notes

1 Tables showing percentages

The row or column percentages may add to 99% or 101% because of rounding.

The varying positions of the percentage signs and bases in the tables denote the presentation of different types of information. Where there is a percentage sign at the head of a column and the base at the foot, the whole distribution is presented and the individual percentages add to between 99% and 101%. Where there is no percentage sign in the table and a note above the figures, the figures refer to the proportion of people who had the attribute being discussed, and the complementary proportion, to add to 100%, is not shown in the table.

The following conventions have been used within tables showing percentages:

-	no cases
0	values less than 0.5%

2 Small bases

Very small bases have been avoided wherever possible because of the relatively high sampling errors that attach to small numbers. Often where the numbers are not large enough to justify the use of all categories, classifications have been condensed. However, an item within a classification is occasionally shown separately, even though the base is small, because to combine it with another large category would detract from the value of the larger category. In general, percentage distributions are shown if the base is 30 or more. Where the base is slightly lower, actual numbers are shown in square brackets.

3. Significant differences

Care should be taken in interpreting findings presented in this report owing to relatively small bases for the four samples of homeless people. This means that even apparently large differences between and within groups of homeless people may not be statistically significant.

Summary of main findings

This report presents the results from the OPCS Survey of Psychiatric Morbidity among homeless people. The survey covered a broad range of people who do not have adequate shelter who were defined according to their accommodation circumstances:

- Residents of hostels
- Residents of private sector leased and short life accommodation (PSLA)
- Adults staying in nightshelters
- People sleeping rough sampled through day centres

One chapter has been devoted to describing the psychiatric morbidity and associated characteristics of each of these four samples of homeless people: Chapters 5 to 8. At the beginning of each of these chapters, there is a summary of the survey results for the particular group of homeless people under discussion. In this summary, data from all four chapters are brought together to compare their characteristics. Care should be taken in interpreting findings presented in this summary and the main body of the report owing to the relatively small sample sizes. This means that even apparently large differences between groups may not be statistically significant.

Personal characteristics

Whereas men predominated in hostels, nightshelters and day centres, women were more likely to be staying in private sector leased accommodation than men. These women tended to be different from other homeless adults in that many were part of two-parent or one-parent homeless families rather than single homeless people.

Just less than 20% of the sample of homeless people sleeping rough who used day centres were aged 16-24 compared with around 30% of residents of hostels and nightshelters and nearly 40% of those in private sector leased accommodation.

In the survey very few people who were interviewed in day centres or nightshelters were from ethnic minorities, whereas 24% of hostel residents and 44% of those in private sector leased accommodation identified themselves as being from non-White ethnic groups.

About half the people in all four samples had no qualifications; a similar proportion were economically inactive.

Prevalence of psychiatric morbidity

The prevalence of neurotic disorders among residents of hostels and PSLA was very similar, 38% and 35% respectively, around two and a half times the proportion among people living in private households.

The prevalence of psychosis was estimated to be 2% among residents of PSLA, and 8% among hostel residents.

For the homeless people sampled in nightshelters and day centres, prevalence rates of neurosis and psychosis were not obtainable. However, after the administration of the GHQ12, about 6 in 10 of both groups had scores at or above the threshold of psychiatric caseness, ie 4 or more.

Information to measure alcohol and drug dependence was obtained for all four samples. The lowest level of alcohol dependence, 3%, was among the PSLA sample, a group which has a large proportion of women many of whom had dependent children. Whereas 16% of hostel residents were defined as alcohol dependent, the proportions among nightshelter residents and day centre visitors were considerably greater at 44% and 50% respectively.

The measure of drug dependence used on the survey was based on regularity of use and is not very robust with regard to cannabinoid drugs. The prevalence of dependence on non-cannabinoid drugs rose from 2% and 6% among PSLA and hostel residents respectively, to 13% among those using day centres and 22% of those living in nightshelters.

Use of alcohol, drugs and tobacco

Looking at alcohol consumption, rather than dependence, considerable variation was again found between the samples. Very heavy drinking (defined as a weekly consumption of over 50 units of alcohol for men and over 35 units for women) was recorded for 3% of PSLA residents, 14% of hostel residents and around 40% of those living in nightshelters and those sleeping rough using day centres.

A similar trend was found when looking at drug use, the proportions using any drug, cannabis or non-cannabinoids, ranged from 16% of PSLA residents, to 25% of hostel dwellers, rising to 37% of day centre visitors and 46% of homeless people staying in nightshelters.

The majority of homeless people smoked cigarettes; many smoked heavily, at least 20 a day. People sleeping rough had the biggest proportion of heavy smokers, 46% closely followed by nightshelter residents at 43%. The proportion of heavy smokers among hostel residents, at 34%, was practically double that of tenants of PSLA, 18%. The corresponding proportion among people living in private households was 11%.

The prevalence of very heavy drinking, drug use or heavy smoking varied by significant neurotic psychopathology (based on the CIS-R) or psychiatric caseness (based on the GHQ12).

The two most notable differences were that 28% of PSLA residents with neurosis were heavy smokers compared with 12% of their non-neurotic counterparts; 36% of hostel residents with neurosis were drug users compared with 18% of the non-neurotic group. No difference was apparent for the use of all three substances according to psychiatric caseness among the sample sleeping rough.

Long-standing illness, treatment and use of services

When residents were asked whether they had a limiting long-standing illness, about 4 in 10 residents of PSLA reported some disorder compared with 5 in 10 of those living in hostels and nightshelters and 6 in 10 of homeless people visiting day centres. In all samples a physical illness was more frequently reported than a mental illness. Those with significant neurotic psychopathology (based on the CIS-R) or psychiatric caseness (based on the GHQ12) were far more likely to report a long-standing illness. Among PSLA, hostel and nightshelter residents between 60-62% of cases reported any illness compared with 24-37% of non-cases. The difference for homeless people sleeping rough was far less: 68% of cases and 52% of non-cases reported an illness.

Between 63% and 73% of those in each sample had consulted a GP within the 12 months prior to interview. Hostel residents with a neurotic disorder had the largest proportion of GP attenders, 85%, whereas among those sleeping rough with a GHQ12 score of less than 4, just over half, 53%, had seen a GP in the past 12 months. Across the four groups of homeless people, there was a remarkable similarity in the proportion who had received secondary care services (in-patient stay and outpatient visit) in the past year, about 56%.

In night shelters and day centres, 11-12% of respondents were prescribed hypnotics or anxiolytics. Antidepressants were taken by 2-5% of all respondents.

Economic activity and financial circumstances

Not surprisingly, the vast majority of homeless people in the survey were either unemployed or economically inactive This latter group consisted of two main categories: those permanently unable to work and others looking after their families - the latter group were predominantly women living in private sector leased accommodation. The proportions who said they were permanently unable to work represented 18% of nightshelter residents, 19% of hostel residents and 24% of those sleeping rough visiting day centres.

The relative lack of employment of homeless people was reflected in their financial situation in that between two-thirds and three quarters of all homeless people were in receipt of state benefits. Just looking at Income Support, 51% of PSLA residents were receiving this State benefit as were 58% of homeless people sleeping rough, and 64% and 68% of hostel and nightshelter residents respectively.

Social functioning and stressful life events

Information on these two topics was only collected for PSLA and hostel residents. Poor social integration, assessed by having 3 or fewer people in one's primary support group, was found for 16% of those living in private sector leased accommodation and 22% of hostel residents. In both cases, the proportions of residents with poor social functioning was greater among the neurotic than the non-neurotic group: 27% compared with 19% (PSLA) and 28% compared with 9% (hostels).

Forty one percent of PSLA tenants and forty five percent of hostel residents had experienced at least two stressful life events in the six months prior to interview. In each sample the proportion having had two such events in the neurotic group was about twice that of the non-neurotic group: 61% compared with 29% (PSLA) and 65% compared with 32% (hostels).

1 Background, aims and coverage of the survey

1.1 Background

Mental illness was identified as one of the five key areas for action in 'The Health of the Nation', a White Paper published by the Department of Health in July 1992.[1] The main target in this area was to improve significantly the health and social functioning of people with mental illness. To achieve this goal, it is necessary to have good baseline information about mental illness. In 1992, the Department of Health in conjunction with the Scottish Office and the Welsh Office, commissioned OPCS to carry out a survey of psychiatric morbidity. The OPCS survey is the first nationally representative survey of psychiatric morbidity to be carried out in Great Britain and covers homeless people, residents of institutions catering for mentally ill people, and people living in private households.

Previous research among homeless people has shown that there is a particularly high prevalence of major psychiatric morbidity in this group - estimates vary from 30% to 50%.[2] Schizophrenia was the most commonly found disorder and alcohol and drug misuse have also been found to be significant problems. However, these studies have tended to concentrate on a small number of hostels or shelters, or are based on studies of adults of no fixed abode visiting hospitals. Most have concentrated on single homeless people. Because these studies used different methodologies to assess mental disorder, it is difficult to generalise from their findings.

OPCS was therefore commissioned to extend the private household survey of psychiatric morbidity to cover the homeless population. This report presents results from the homeless survey. Previous reports have presented results for other population groups.

Two distinctive features of this survey were:

(a) taking a representative sample of homeless adults, covering a large number of establishments where homeless people are found, including both single homeless people and families.

(b) asking the same questions as in the other parts of the survey programme in a standardised way and recording answers in the same systematic manner.

1.2 Aims of the survey

There were three main aims of the survey:

Prevalence

One of the main reasons for carrying out this survey was to estimate the prevalence of psychiatric morbidity according to diagnostic category among homeless adults aged 16 to 64 years in Great Britain.

Service use, medication and treatment

The varying use of services and the receipt of care are examined in relation to psychiatric morbidity. Information is given on services provided under the Care Programme Approach, and about the receipt of health services through hostels and centres for homeless people as well as other mainstream health services.

Lifestyle indicators

Another principal aim was to estimate the extent of alcohol and drug dependence and to describe the relationship between mental disorders and drinking, drug use and smoking.

Other topics of interest

In addition, data were collected to enable the survey to:

- show relationships between physical complaints and psychiatric morbidity

- examine the social isolation associated with mental disorder

- investigate how major events in the previous six months were related to how people were feeling at the time of the interview

- compare the employment and finances of adults according to mental disorder.

1.3 Coverage of the survey

Region

The population which was surveyed comprised adults living in England, Wales and Scotland (excluding the Highlands and Islands) who were homeless according to the definitions given below.

Age

The survey focused on the prevalence of psychiatric morbidity among adults aged 16 to 64. Adults aged 65 or above were excluded because specialised interviewing and assessment procedures would be required. Although there is increased interest in the circumstances of children in homeless families, this was beyond the remit of the present study. Surveys of homeless children require specialised sampling, interviewing and assessment procedures.

Definition of homelessness

The survey was interested in a broad range of people who do not have adequate shelter who could be defined according to their accommodation circumstances.

A   Residents of hostels
B   Residents of private sector leased and short life accommodation
C   Adults staying in nightshelters
D   People sleeping rough sampled through day centres

Group A - Residents of hostels

The survey covered a wide range of hostels in both the statutory and the voluntary and private sector. Examples of hostels which were included are those run by the Salvation Army, YMCA, DSS Resettlement Agency and hostels for people with alcohol or drugs problems. Hostels varied in the degree of staff support, services and facilities they offered, the client groups they targeted, and the length of stay permitted.

Hostels which catered specifically for people with mental health problems were excluded as they were covered in the institutional survey. Hostels for students or working people only were also excluded.

Group B - Residents of private sector leased and short life accommodation (PSLA)

Local authorities have developed a large stock of property leased from landlords in the private sector. By the end of June 1993, approximately 24,300 households were placed in temporary PSL accommodation by local authorities in England.[3] The use of PSLA as a substitute for bed and breakfast and hotel accommodation (B&B) led to a considerable fall in the number of households in B&B accommodation; at the end of June 1993 around 6,000 households were temporarily accommodated in B&B. The survey reflected this by covering PSL accommodation but excluding bed and breakfast and hotel accommodation. PSL accommodation is predominantly used to house statutory homeless households, that is those who are considered to be in priority need under the homelessness provisions of the housing legislation. These are mainly families and pregnant women, but do include some vulnerable people with mental illness.

Group C - Adults staying in nightshelters

The survey included nightshelters as a sub-group of hostels. Although some residents of nightshelters stay for a considerable length of time, they are generally more transient than the residents of other types of hostel and consequently a different methodology was required in nightshelters.

A resident of a nightshelter was defined as anyone present on the night the sample was drawn. Some nightshelter residents sleep rough intermittently and, as such, they may also have been eligible for the survey in day centres.

Group D - People sleeping rough using day centres

There are no accurate estimates of the numbers of people sleeping rough and the population itself is continually changing. Official estimates of the size of this population from the 1991 Census enumeration was 2,827 people at known sites in Great Britain.[4] Other sources give higher figures. Shelter, the national campaign for homeless people, suggest that up to 8,600 people are sleeping rough in England.[5] These estimates are based on DSS statistics for people receiving Income Support who had no accommodation at the end of May 1991.

The difficulty in getting accurate estimates of the number of people sleeping rough causes problems in drawing a representative sample. For this survey, people who sleep rough were sampled through their use of day centres for homeless people as a practical and cost-effective alternative to sampling in open places. It was also considered inappropriate to conduct this survey while people used soup runs because of the interview length and subject matter. Adults who sleep rough but do not use day centres were therefore excluded from the survey although it is likely that their characteristics were similar to those of adults included in the survey. A study of single homeless people conducted for the Department of Environment[6] showed no significant health differences among people who slept rough between those who were sampled in day centres and those sampled at soup runs; the proportions who reported that they suffered depression, anxiety or nerves were 37% and 43% respectively.

As in the DoE survey, only people who had slept rough on at least one of the past seven nights were included in this part of the survey. The term 'sleeping rough' includes sleeping in make-shift shelters and tents.

This survey did not attempt to cover other groups of homeless people such as the 'hidden homeless', that is, people who would like to have their own housing but are forced to share accommodation.

Season

Interviewing took place between July and August 1994. It is known that there is some seasonal variation in where homeless people stay, for example, adults who stay in nightshelters in the winter may sleep rough in the summer. Since the survey included both the nightshelter population and people who slept rough, it was not necessary for fieldwork to cover both seasons.

1.4 Coverage of the current report

The main purpose of this Report is to present prevalence rates of psychiatric morbidity among adults aged 16 to 64 in Great Britain in the four groups of homeless people covered by the survey. In order to interpret these results, it is important to have an understanding of the conceptual approach and methods adopted for this study, and these are described in Chapters 2 and 3.

Because little is currently known about homeless people Chapter 4 presents the characteristics of adults in the four samples covered. The main results on psychiatric morbidity are given for each sample separately in Chapters 5 to 8. Each of these chapters consists of 2 parts. The first is concerned with the prevalence of psychiatric morbidity and includes alcohol and drug dependence. The second part examines the lifestyle indicators such as alcohol and drug use, physical health, the use of medication and treatment, and of health, social and voluntary care services in relation to psychiatric morbidity. In the second part, comparisons are made between adults with a neurotic disorder and those with no neurotic disorder. Adults with a psychotic disorder are omitted from these analyses owing to the very different nature of their mental illness.

The purpose of the commentary in this report is to present a descriptive account of the key findings and main differences observed between adults with psychiatric morbidity and other adults. Sampling errors have not been calculated because of their complexity but they are known to be relatively large owing to the small sample sizes. Consequently, testing for significant differences between figures presented in this report has not been possible. Nevertheless, it is likely that very large differences would be statistically significant even with the small bases. Furthermore, striking findings that would probably not reach statistical significance given small bases, may

still reflect real differences between the groups concerned. Hence, care should be taken in interpreting the data.

Prevalence rates are presented for each sample separately and comparisons are made between samples. However, we have not attempted to produce a single estimate of psychiatric morbidity among all homeless people. This is because the samples are not exclusive; adults may move between hostels, nightshelters and sleeping rough. Even if it were possible to adjust for the overlap between the samples, some of the population sizes cannot be estimated with accuracy in order to produce a combined prevalence rate. Furthermore, the survey covers 4 groups of homeless people which, together, do not form a comprehensive sample of all homeless people, so a combined prevalence rate would be of limited applicability.

1.5 Other reports in the series on psychiatric morbidity

This is the seventh of eight reports on the four surveys on psychiatric morbidity and deals exclusively with the results of the survey of homeless people. Bulletin 3 which is published contemporaneously presents a summary of the main findings on the prevalence of psychiatric morbidity which are found in this report.

The full set of results from the OPCS survey of psychiatric morbidity are presented in a series of eight reports and four bulletins published in 1995 and 1996. The content of these reports and bulletins are summarised below in the order of the publication schedule.

Private household survey

Bulletin No.1 *(Published 1994)*
Prevalence of psychiatric morbidity

Report 1 *(Published 1995)*
Prevalence of psychiatric morbidity by socio-demographic correlates; co-morbidity among psychiatric disorders.

Report 2 *(Published 1996)*
Characteristics of people with mental disorders, medication and other forms of treatment, service use, and patient satisfaction with treatment and services.

Report 3 *(Published 1996)*
Difficulties associated with mental disorders in respect of activities of daily living, employment, social functioning and finances. Recent stressful life events and lifestyle behaviours (use of tobacco, alcohol and drugs and their consequences).

Institutions survey

Bulletin No.2 *(Published 1995)*
Prevalence of psychiatric morbidity in institutions.

Report 4 *(Published 1996)*
Prevalence of psychiatric morbidity by type of institution; co-occurrence of psychiatric disorders.

Report 5 *(Published 1996)*
Characteristics of people with mental disorders living in institutions, medication, other forms of treatment, and service use within and outside the institution.

Report 6 *(Published 1996)*
Difficulties associated with mental disorders in respect of activities of daily living, employment and finances, social functioning, and the use of alcohol, drugs and tobacco.

Survey of homeless people

Bulletin No.3 *(Published 1996)*
Prevalence of psychiatric morbidity among homeless people.

Report 7 *(Published 1996)*
Prevalence of psychiatric morbidity by type of 'accommodation'; medication, other forms of treatment, and service use; difficulties

associated with mental disorders in respect of housing, employment, social functioning, and finances. Recent stressful life events and lifestyle behaviours (use of tobacco, alcohol and drugs and their consequences).

People suffering from a psychotic illness

Bulletin No.4 *(Published 1996)*
Summary of the characteristics of people with psychosis living in private households, recognised lodgings and group homes.

Report 8 *(Published 1996)*
Profiles of people with psychosis in terms of differential use of treatment and services.

Access to the data

Anonymised data from all four surveys will be lodged with the ESRC Data Archive, University of Essex, within 3 months of the publication of the final main report.[7]

Notes and references

1. *The Health of the Nation: A Strategy for Health in England*, DH, HMSO, 1992

2. Scott J, (1993) Review article: Homelessness and mental illness, *British Journal of Psychiatry*; **162**: 314-25

3. DoE, December 1993 *Information Bulletin 849: Households found accommodation under the homelessness provisions of the 1985 Housing Act: England, Statistics for the third quarter of 1993*, Tables 4a and 5

4. OPCS. *1991 Census Preliminary report for England and Wales: Supplementary Monitor on people sleeping rough* (1991)

5. Mann J, Smith A.(1993) *Who says there's no housing problem?* Shelter report (2nd Edition), pp 11-12.

6. DoE. Single Homeless People, HMSO (1993)

7. Independent researchers who wish to carry out their own analyses should apply to the Archive for access. For further information about archived data, please contact:

   Ms Kathy Sayer
   ESRC Data Archive
   University of Essex
   Wivenhoe Park
   Colchester
   Essex CO4 3SQ

   Tel: (UK) 01206 872323
   FAX: (UK) 01206 872003
   Email: archive@:Essex.AC.UK.

2 Definitions of terms and their measurement

2.1 Introduction

For this Report we have tried to carry out similar analysis on each of the four groups of homeless people. The concepts on which the analysis is based, which cover measures of psychiatric disorders, alcohol and drug dependence as well as social and economic indicators are described here rather than repeating them in each chapter. A description of the four categories of homeless people can be found in Chapter 1.

2.2 Assessment of psychiatric disorders

Assessment of neurotic psychopathology

Two methods were used to assess and classify neurotic disorders among homeless people depending on the sample in which they were identified. For homeless people resident in hostels or living in private sector leased accommodation, the principal instrument used to assess neurotic disorders was the revised Clinical Interview Schedule (CIS-R).[1] For residents of nightshelters and people sleeping rough using day centres, the GHQ12 was employed.[2] Although we would have liked to ask the CIS-R of everyone, pilot studies showed that this instrument was inappropriate when interviewing time was severely restricted. A relatively short and easily administered questionnaire was required for users of nightshelters and day centres owing to respondents' short periods of concentration and the desire of staff to meet the needs of people who use their premises and facilities. The GHQ12 was, in fact, also asked of hostel residents and those in private sector leased accommodation but this was mainly to investigate the GHQ12 scores in relation to CIS-R scores (see Appendix C).

The CIS-R

The Revised Clinical Interview Schedule (CIS-R) establishes the existence of a particular neurotic symptom in the past month and leads the interviewer on to further enquiry giving a more detailed assessment of the symptom **in the past week**: frequency, duration, severity and time since onset. Algorithms are applied to the data to delineate six types of neurotic disorder.

The CIS-R is made up of 14 sections, each section covering a particular area of neurotic symptoms.

The 14 Sections of the CIS-R

Somatic symptoms
Fatigue
Concentration and forgetfulness
Sleep problems
Irritability
Worry about physical health
Depression
Depressive ideas
Worry
Anxiety
Phobias
Panic
Compulsions
Obsessions

Each section within the interview schedule starts with a variable number of mandatory questions which can be regarded as sift or filter questions. They establish the existence of a particular neurotic symptom in the past month. A positive response to these questions leads the interviewer on to further enquiry giving a more detailed assessment of the symptom **in the past week**: frequency, duration, severity and time since onset. It is the answers to these questions which determine the informant's score on each section. More frequent and more severe symptoms result in higher scores.

The minimum score on each section is 0, where the symptom was either not present in the past week or was present only in mild degree. The maximum score on each section is 4 (except for the section on Depressive Ideas which has a maximum score of 5).

- Summed scores from all 14 sections range between 0 and 57.

- The overall threshold score for significant psychiatric morbidity is 12.

- Symptoms are regarded as significant if they have a score of 2 or more.

The elements which contribute to a score are shown in Appendix B, Part 1. As an illustration, the elements which contribute to a score on the section on Anxiety are shown below.

Calculation of symptom score for Anxiety from the CIS-R

                                                          Score
Felt **generally** anxious/nervous/ tense for **4 days or more** in the past seven days.......................1

In past seven days anxiety /nervousness/tension has been **very unpleasant**...........................1

In the past seven days have felt **any of the following symptoms** when anxious/nervous/tense (Racing heart, sweating or shaking hands, feeling dizzy, difficulty getting one's breath, dry mouth, butterflies in stomach, nausea or wanting to vomit) 1

Felt anxious/nervous/tense for **more than three hours** in total on any one of the past seven days.................1

Any combination of the elements produce the section score.

For purposes of analysis overall CIS-R scores have been grouped into six categories: 0-5, 6-11, 12-17, 18-23, 24-29 and 30 or above, or into two categories indicating those below threshold, 0-11, or at or above the threshold score, 12 or above.

Diagnoses are obtained by looking at the answers to various sections, including questions which do not necessarily score points. After applying algorithms based on ICD-10 diagnostic criteria, six neurotic disorders were identified.[3]

- Generalised Anxiety Disorder (GAD)
- Depressive episode
- Mixed anxiety and depressive disorder
- Phobia
- Obsessive-Compulsive Disorder (OCD)
- Panic disorder

The algorithms for all disorders are shown in Appendix B. It should be noted that social impairment is included in the algorithms for depressive episode, phobia and Obsessive-Compulsive Disorder, assessed by one question relating to all significant neurotic symptoms (see Schedule A, section O). An example of an algorithm is shown below, for Generalised Anxiety Disorder.

Algorithm for Generalised Anxiety Disorder (GAD)

Conditions which must apply are:

- Duration greater than six months
- Free-floating anxiety
- Autonomic overactivity
- Overall score on Anxiety section was 2 or more

The GHQ12

The General Health Questionnaire (GHQ) was designed to be a self-administered screening test aimed at detecting psychiatric disorders among respondents in community and non-psychiatric clinical settings. The 12 question version, (GHQ12) has many advantages for use among homeless people: easy to administer, fairly short and acceptable to respondents.

To the extent that an individual's score on the GHQ12 gives an assessment of their position on a continuum from normality to undoubted illness, it can be thought of as giving a probability estimate of that person being a psychiatric 'case'.

The GHQ12, reproduced in Appendix D, concerns itself with two major classes of phenomena: inability to carry out 'normal healthy functions' and the appearance of new phenomena of a distressing nature. The GHQ12 asks respondents about their health **over the past few weeks**.

An individual can have a GHQ12 score ranging from 0 to 12. In order to present results comparing high scorers with low scorers, it is necessary to decide upon a threshold score. Previous studies, reviewed by Goldberg (1988) have used scores ranging from 2 to 4. In this survey, the score of 4 was chosen as the threshold as this was shown from our comparative analysis (see Appendix C) to be closest to the threshold for the CIS-R; a score of 4 or more on the GHQ12 is deemed to equate to a score of 12 or more on the CIS-R.

Assessment of psychotic psychopathology

The approach used to assess psychotic psychopathology was the same for the four samples of homeless people.

Making assessments of psychotic rather than neurotic disorders is more problematic for lay interviewers. A structured questionnaire is too restrictive and a semi-structured questionnaire requires the use of clinical judgements.

Therefore OPCS interviewers were only asked to carry out an initial, general investigation: was there any possibility of the subject suffering from a psychotic illness? If further investigation was needed, psychiatrists were asked to carry out a follow-up clinical interview. The questions for the initial investigation were pitched at such a level to reduce as far as possible the number of false negatives albeit at the cost of increasing the false positive rate.

The sift for presently occurring symptoms, Psychosis Sift Questionnaire (PSQ), was developed specifically for this project.[4] In addition, informants were asked directly what was the matter with them; whether they were taking anti-psychotic drugs or having anti-psychotic injections, and whether they had contact with any health care professional for a mental, nervous or emotional problem which had been labelled as a psychotic illness. These additional questions were added to minimise the false negative rate in the context of a disorder of low prevalence.

Clinicians who followed up potential cases were trained to carry out their interviews using SCAN (Schedules for Clinical Assessment in Neuropsychiatry) which is programmed on to a laptop computer.[5] SCAN is a set of instruments aimed at assessing, measuring and classifying the psychopathology and behaviour associated with the major psychiatric disorders of adult life. Of its four main components, the PSE10 was the one deemed most applicable for the purposes of this survey.[6] The PSE10 itself has two parts. Part One covers, inter alia, anxiety, depressive and bipolar disorders. Part Two includes the psychotic disorders of interest to the survey: schizophrenia, delusional and schizoaffective disorders, plus mania and affective bipolar disorder.

Because of the logistical difficulties in following up a mobile population throughout Great Britain with a psychiatric assessment, not everyone eligible for a SCAN interview was contacted. When a SCAN interview was done, those who were assessed as having psychosis in the past year were defined for this survey as a 'definite' case of psychosis. If a SCAN interview was not done but the person screened positive in the OPCS interview because of self-reported psychosis or being prescribed antipsychotic medication, the OPCS survey data were reviewed. This involved collating coded responses and verbatim answers to create case studies. The topics included in this review were:

- age and sex of the subject
- subject's report of longstanding illness and onset of episode
- doctor's diagnosis of a mental, nervous or emotional problem as reported by the informant
- the subject's medication (including injections), dosage and compliance
- psychotic symptoms (as measured by the Psychosis Screening Questionnaire)
- CIS-R scores (if available) and GHQ12 scores
- Measures of alcohol and drug dependence (for residents of nightshelters and those using day centres)

- Use of mental health services (for residents of nightshelters and those using day centres)

Two clinically experienced psychiatric epidemiologists working independently were sent all the case studies for assessment. Based on this information they ascribed a diagnosis of psychosis with an indicator of certainty. Overall there was very good agreement between the assessors. If the subject was on antipsychotic medication, with an appropriate dosage, and the doctor was reported to have given a diagnosis of psychosis, this was defined as psychosis with higher certainty than in other cases where the assessment was just based on one fact relating to medication or what the subject said was the matter with them. If subjects only screened positive for psychosis because of the response to the Psychosis Screening Questionnaire, they were regarded as having a low likelihood of psychosis. This was based on evidence from the private household survey and borne out by results of SCAN interviews on the homeless survey.

Type of assessment	Applicability	Outcome
SCAN	Adults who screened positive for psychosis, with a SCAN positive result for psychosis	Definite
Case study	Adults who screened positive for psychosis (excluding those solely identified by the PSQ) who were SCAN negative for psychosis or did not have a SCAN interview	Almost certain or Fairly certain or Little certainty or Definitely not psychotic
No assessment	Adults who screened positive for psychosis solely identified by the PSQ	Very low likelihood assumed to be non-psychotic
	Adults who screened negative for psychosis	Definitely not psychotic

For consistency even those who were found not to have a psychotic illness after a SCAN interview were assessed as case studies. In a small number of these cases, the assessment of the case study indicated the presence of psychosis.

A summary of assessment procedures, the conditions for their applicability, and the range of consequences for each assessment is presented on page 10. Only the three outcomes - definite, almost certain and fairly certain - are deemed to define cases of psychosis to be used in calculating prevalence rates.

2.3 Definitions and measures of social indicators

Social functioning

This survey considered two aspects of social functioning: social networks and involvement in social and leisure activities at clubs or centres. Data were only collected for hostel residents and those living in private sector leased accommodation.

i) Extent of social networks

In this survey information about social networks focused on the numbers of friends and relatives (aged 16 and over) respondents felt close to.

Data were collected about several groups of people:

- adult family members living with the respondent
- adults who lived with respondents that respondents felt close to, including staff living on the premises
- relatives who did not live with respondents that they felt close to
- friends or acquaintances who did not live with respondents that would be described as close or good friends.

Close friends and relatives form an individual's 'primary support group'. Previous research has suggested that adults with a total primary support group of 3 people or fewer are at greatest risk of psychiatric morbidity.[7][8]

ii) Attendance at clubs

Information is presented about residents' attendance at four specific types of place for social activities, some catering specifically for adults those with mental health problems.

Use of alcohol, drugs and tobacco

Measures of alcohol use, drug misuse, and cigarette smoking are available for residents who had personal interviews.

Drug misuse includes the use of illegal drugs such as cannabis, stimulants and hallucinogens, and the extra-medical use of some prescription medicines. The consumption of prescribed medication in general is covered in a separate section of each chapter.

Obtaining information about people's drinking, drug-taking and cigarette smoking is difficult, for example, social surveys of the general population consistently record lower levels of alcohol consumption than would be expected from alcohol sales. This is for a variety of reasons, such as non-deliberate underestimation (for example of amounts drunk at home) and, particularly regarding drug misuse, due to respondents' concerns about confidentiality. However, it is not known whether, or to what extent, similar problems occur with regard to data collected on homeless people.

i) Alcohol consumption

The methodology used on this survey to categorise alcohol consumption is the same as that used in the OPCS Survey of Psychiatric Morbidity among adults living in private households[9], the General Household Survey (GHS)[10] and the 1993 Health Survey for England[11].

Informants were asked how often they had drunk each of the following five types of drink in the previous year and how much of each type they usually drank on any one day:

Shandy (excluding bottles/cans with very low alcohol content)
Beer, lager, stout, cider
Spirits or liqueurs
Sherry or martini
Wine

Informants described their consumption in terms of standard measures which contained similar amounts of alcohol, one unit of alcohol being approximately equivalent to a half pint of beer, a single measure of spirits (1/6 gill), a glass of wine (about 4.5 fluid ounces) or a small glass of sherry or fortified wine (2 fluid ounces).

The alcohol consumption rating is calculated by multiplying the number of units of each type of drink consumed on a 'usual' day by a conversion factor relating to the frequency with which it was drunk, and totalling across all drinks:

Multiplying factors for converting drinking frequency and number of units consumed on a usual day into a number of units consumed per week.

Drinking frequency	Multiplying factor	
Almost every day	7.0	
5 or 6 times per week	5.5	
3 or 4 times per week	3.5	
Once or twice per week	1.5	
Once or twice per month	0.375	(1.5/4)
Once or twice per 6 months	0.058	(1.5/26)
Once or twice per year	0.029	(1.5/52)

When the survey took place in 1994 the recommended sensible drinking levels were 21 units per week for men and 14 for women. Although these levels were increased at the end of 1995, analysis of the data in this report is based on the 1994 guidelines to retain comparability with the data from the private household survey and the General Household Survey. Thus, residents who are described as being 'Fairly heavy' 'Heavy' or 'Very heavy' drinkers were consuming over the recommended sensible level of alcohol when the survey took place. The way in which the descriptive labels used in the tables relate to units of alcohol is shown below:

Alcohol consumption categories, based on usual weekly consumption (units) over the previous 12 months

	Men	Women
Abstainer in the past year	Informant drank no alcohol	
Occasional drinker	Under 1 unit per week	
	(units per week)	
Light	1 - 10	1 - 7
Moderate	11 - 21	8 - 14

Over the recommended sensible level:

	Men	Women
Fairly heavy	22 - 35	15 - 25
Heavy	36 - 50	26 - 35
Very heavy	51 or more	36 or more

One of the particular problems of measuring alcohol consumption among homeless people is that this population contains many heavy drinkers, and from time to time individuals may be in a period of detoxification; stopping drinking for health reasons. Alcohol consumption and dependence was only assessed for those currently drinking. Further caution is required in interpreting consumption measures because of memory problems and defining average amounts. People drank alcohol when they had money to buy it. Despite these caveats, alcohol consumption level is likely to be fairly robust in identifying categories of very heavy drinking.

ii) Alcohol dependence

Three aspects of alcohol dependence were assessed; loss of control, symptomatic behaviour and binge drinking. Twelve questions were taken from the 1984 US National Alcohol Survey. [12]

Informants were classified as alcohol dependent if they responded positively to three or more of the following twelve statements:

Loss of control

1. Once I started drinking it was difficult for me to stop before I became completely drunk.

2. I sometimes kept on drinking after I had promised myself not to.

3. I deliberately tried to cut down or stop drinking, but I was unable to do so.

4. Sometimes I needed a drink so badly that I could not think of anything else.

Symptomatic behaviour

5. I have skipped a number of regular meals while drinking.

6. I have often had an alcoholic drink the first thing when I got up.

7. I have had a strong drink in the morning to get over the previous night's drinking.

8. I have woken up the next day not being able to remember some of the things I had done while drinking.

9. My hands shook a lot in the morning after drinking.

10. I need more alcohol than I used to, to get the same effect as before.

11. Sometimes I have woken up during the night or early morning sweating all over because of drinking.

Binge drinking

12. I have stayed drunk for several days at a time.

Adults were defined as having 'loss of control' or 'symptomatic behaviour' if they responded positively to 2 or more of the relevant statements and those who responded positively to the statement on binge drinking were defined as 'binge drinkers'. However, adults who satisfied the conditions for any one of these three components may not have met the criteria for being defined as alcohol dependent.

The private household survey also considered 'alcohol problems'. However, corresponding data were not collected in this survey as many of the questions were not appropriate for homeless people.

iii) Drug use

Information on drug use was obtained from responses to a self-completion questionnaire asked of all survey respondents. Informants were asked about their use of drugs including sedatives, tranquillisers, cannabis, amphetamines, cocaine, opiates, hallucinogens, Ecstasy and solvents. The medical use of prescribed drugs, most usually sedatives and tranquillisers is analysed separately.

Extra-medical and illicit use of drugs was ascertained by presenting informants with a list of drugs and asking if they had used any of these without a prescription, or more than was prescribed for them, or to get high. Sedatives and tranquillisers were placed highest on the list to deter adults who did not use illicit drugs but did misuse medication from assuming the questions did not apply to them.

List of commonly used drugs

Sleeping pills, Barbiturates, Sedatives, Downers, Seconal

Tranquillisers, Valium, Lithium

Cannabis, Marijuana, Hash, Dope, Grass, Ganja, Kif

Amphetamines, Speed, Uppers, Stimulants, Qat

Cocaine, Coke, Crack

Heroin, Smack

Opiates other than heroin: Demerol, Morphine, Methadone, Darvon, Opium, DF118

Psychedelics, Hallucinogens: LSD, Mescaline, Acid, Peyote, Psilocybin (magic) mushrooms

Ecstasy

Solvents, Inhalants, Glue, Amyl nitrate

The questions on drug use and the drug categories were drawn from the drugs section of the Diagnostic Interview Schedule (DIS)[13] and were used in the U.S. ECA study.[14] Questions on injecting drugs and needle sharing were added.

Informants who reported using any of the drugs listed either without a prescription, or at more than the prescribed dosage, or to get high, were then asked if they had taken the drug more than five times in their life. Those who had done so and had also taken the drug in the past twelve months were defined as **users** of the drug.

iv) Drug dependence

Individuals who were defined as users of a drug were classified as dependent on that drug if they reported using it every day for two weeks or more in the past 12 months. This definition is limited in not taking into account amounts of the drug actually consumed, and the effects of drug-taking, or not-taking on the individual. In the self-completion booklet it was not possible to probe for more details about these issues.

It is likely that our definition of drug dependence classified more people as dependent on drugs than a more stringent definition would have done. This is particularly likely with regard to cannabis, where regular users may well not show additional symptoms of dependence. We can be more confident that those using hard drugs every day for 2 weeks or more in the past 12 months would actually be found to be dependent on those drugs had we been able to collect more information.

v) Cigarette smoking

All informants, except proxies, were asked if they had ever smoked cigarettes, cigars or a pipe and if they smoked cigarettes nowadays. If they did smoke, they were asked questions about average daily consumption. Adults were grouped into categories, depending on whether they had ever smoked, and the average daily amount smoked. These categories were identical to those in the 1992 General Household Survey (GHS)[15] and the 1993 Health Survey for England[16], although neither of these surveys covered homeless people.

Cigarette smoking categories

Never regularly smoked
Ex-smokers
Current smokers:
Light	Less than 10 a day
Moderate	Less than 20 a day, but more than 10
Heavy	More than 20 a day

Notes and references

1. Lewis, G., Pelosi, A.J. and Dunn, G., (1992) Measuring Psychiatric disorder in the community: a standardized assessment for use by lay interviewers, *Psychological Medicine*, **22**, 465-486

   Lewis, G. and Pelosi, A. J., *Manual of the Revised Clinical Interview Schedule, (CIS-R)*, June 1990, MRC Institute of Psychiatry

2. Goldberg, D., and Williams, P., (1988) *A Users Guide to the General Health Questionnaire*, NFER-NELSON

3. *The ICD-10 Classification of Mental and Behavioural Disorders: Diagnostic Criteria for Research:* 1993, WHO, Geneva.

4. Bebbington, P.E., and Nayani, T (1995) "The Psychosis Screening Questionnaire" *International Journal of Methods in Psychiatric Research*, **5**: 11-19

5. *Schedules for Clinical Assessment in Neuropsychiatry*, 1992, WHO, Division of Mental Health, Geneva

6. Wing, J. K., et al. "Reliability of the PSE used in a population survey." *Psychological Medicine*, **Vol 7**, 505-516.

7.	Brugha, T.S. et al (1993) The relationship of social network deficits with deficits in social functioning in long-term psychiatric disorders. *Social Psychiatry and Psychiatric Epidemiology,* **28**, 218-224

8.	Brugha et al (1987). The Interview Measure of Social Relationships: the description and evaluation of a survey instrument for assessing personal social resources. *Social Psychiatry,* **22**, 123-128

9.	Meltzer, H., Gill., B, Petticrew, M., and Hinds, K. (1995) *OPCS Surveys of Psychiatric Morbidity in Great Britain, Report 1, The prevalence of psychiatric morbidity among adults living in private households*, HMSO: London

10.	Thomas, M. et al (1994) *1992 General Household Survey.* HMSO, London

11.	Bennett, N. et al (1995) *Health Survey for England 1993.* HMSO, London

12.	Hilton, M. E., (1991) A note on measuring drinking problems in the 1984 National Alcohol Survey in (eds) Clark and Hilton, *Alcohol in America,* State University of New York: Albany

13.	Robins, L. N., Helzer, J. E., Croughan, J. and Ratcliff, K.S., (1981) National Institute of Mental Health Diagnostic Interview Schedule: Its History, Characteristics, and Validity, *Archives of General Psychiatry,* Vol 38, pp 381-389

14.	*Psychiatric Disorders in America, The Epidemiologic Catchment Area Study,* edited by Robins, L. N., and Reiger, D.A., (1991) Free Press, New York

15.	op. cit., Thomas, M. et al (1994)

16.	op cit., Bennett, N, et al (1995)

3   Sampling and interviewing procedures

3.1   Introduction

This chapter describes the creation of sampling frames, the selection of establishments for the survey, the selection of individuals within establishments and the various interviewing procedures which were adopted to maximise response. The survey documents are reproduced in Appendix D.

In the first section of the chapter, the sample designs are presented separately for the four parts of the survey. The second section is concerned with the organisation of the interview in hostels and private sector leased accommodation (PSLA) and then in nightshelters and day centres.

3.2   Sampling procedures

Hostels

A sampling frame of hostels was constructed for the survey from information collected directly from local authority (LA) housing departments. This included hostels for non-statutory homeless people but excluded those which catered solely for adults who were mentally ill, working people or students, those that were known to have no adults aged 16 to 64, and women's refuges. 363 of the 456 housing departments in Great Britain responded to our request for information and 235 reported hostels in their area. These lists were supplemented using known local lists of hostels and those from national organisations which provide hostel accommodation.

44 sample quotas were allocated to 23 of the responding LAs with probability roughly proportional to the hostel population size. Size was initially estimated by the numbers of statutory homeless households placed in

temporary hostel accommodation by LAs, which are produced regularly by the Department of Environment[1], the Scottish Office[2] and the Welsh Office[3]. After the local authorities had been selected, we contacted all the hostels in the area to find out the number of residents aged 16 to 64 to get more accurate estimates of the hostel population size. Some adjustments were then made to the distribution of the sample quota in the selected LAs in order to better reflect these revised estimates.

After hostels were ordered by size within LAs, a systematic equal probability sample of 94 hostels was drawn. Each hostel was assigned a sampling fraction so that the required number of residents would be selected in each LA. Each selected hostel was designated a reserve which interviewers could use as a substitute in the event of a refusal from the hostel or if, despite previous checks, it transpired the hostel was ineligible for the survey.

Interviewers visited the hostels and listed the eligible residents, usually with the help of staff. A resident was eligible for the survey if he or she was aged 16 to 64 and had no other place of residence. Interviewers then drew a systematic sample to select residents. In most cases they used the assigned sampling fraction but, if the hostel was considerably different in size to what was expected, they adjusted the fraction accordingly before they began sampling. In total, 530 adults were interviewed in 92 hostels. *(Figure 3.1)*

PSL accommodation (PSLA)

Although there is no national list of private sector leased and short life accommodation, the numbers of statutory homeless households temporarily placed in such accommodation by local authorities which are regularly produced by the Department of Environment, Scottish

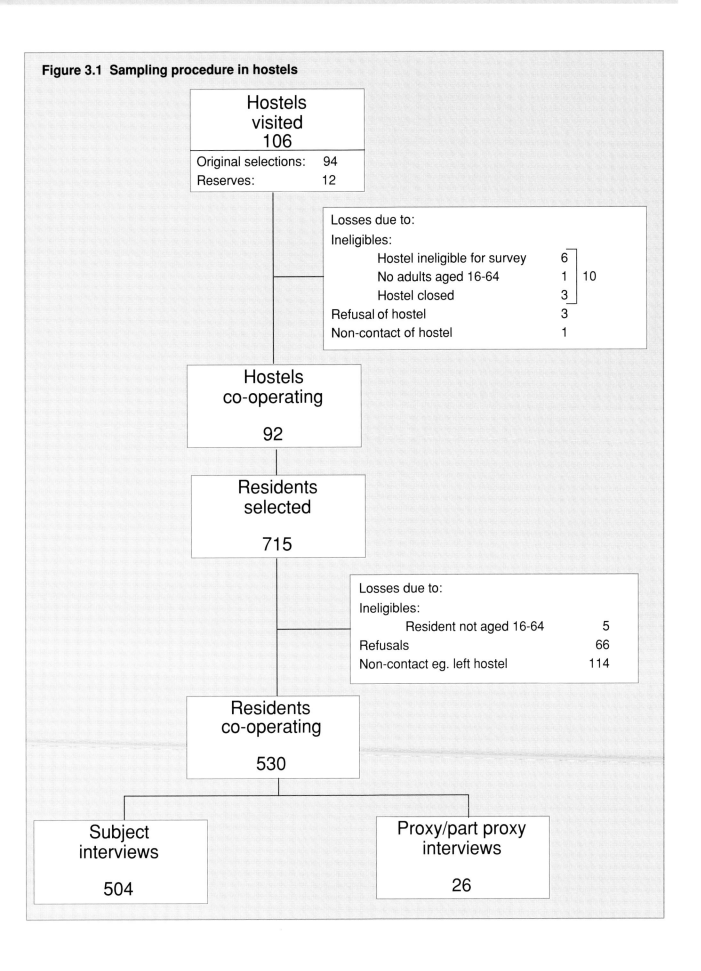

Figure 3.1 Sampling procedure in hostels

Hostels visited 106
Original selections: 94
Reserves: 12

Losses due to:
Ineligibles:
Hostel ineligible for survey 6
No adults aged 16-64 1 } 10
Hostel closed 3
Refusal of hostel 3
Non-contact of hostel 1

Hostels co-operating 92

Residents selected 715

Losses due to:
Ineligibles:
Resident not aged 16-64 5
Refusals 66
Non-contact eg. left hostel 114

Residents co-operating 530

Subject interviews 504

Proxy/part proxy interviews 26

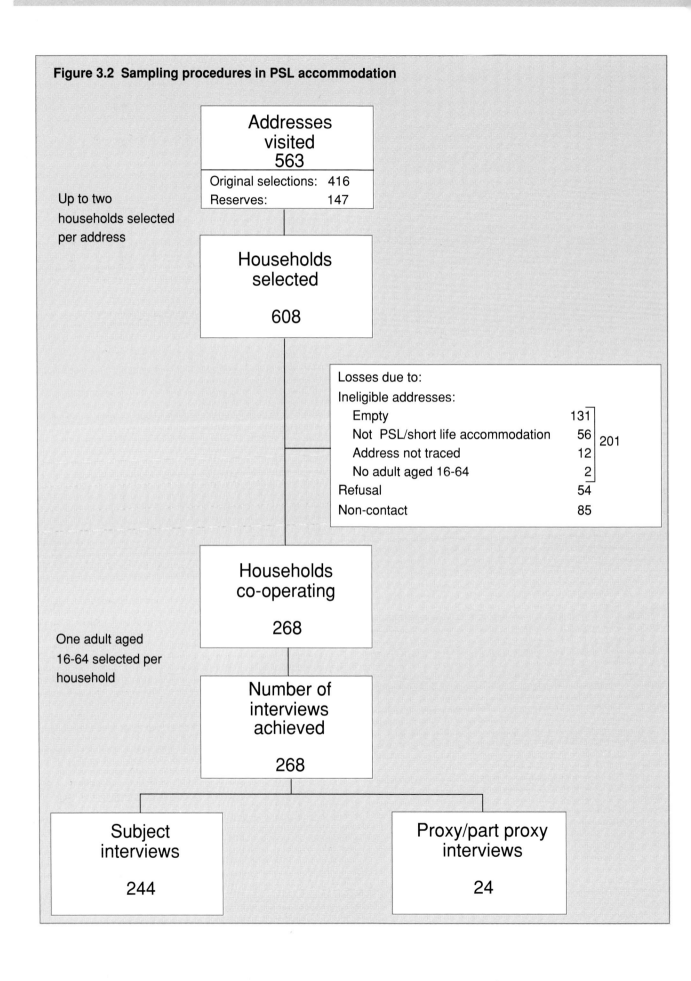

Figure 3.2 Sampling procedures in PSL accommodation

Addresses visited
563
Original selections: 416
Reserves: 147

Up to two households selected per address

Households selected
608

Losses due to:
Ineligible addresses:
Empty 131
Not PSL/short life accommodation 56
Address not traced 12
No adult aged 16-64 2
201
Refusal 54
Non-contact 85

Households co-operating
268

One adult aged 16-64 selected per household

Number of interviews achieved
268

Subject interviews
244

Proxy/part proxy interviews
24

Office and Welsh Office are regarded as a good indicator of the target population size. Information on PSLA was also requested directly from the 456 housing departments in Great Britain. 363 responded and 168 returned details of the number of units of this type of accommodation.

Estimates of the population size from the statutory homeless figures were used to allocate the twenty required sample quotas in approximately representative proportions among the regions of England, and Scotland and Wales. Within the selected regions, sampling quotas were allocated among those local authorities which had responded with details of their PSL accommodation. Twenty quotas were drawn in 15 local authorities; each quota consisted of approximately 23 addresses.

For each quota, addresses were selected systematically from the local authority lists. Each selection was also designated a reserve address which could be used as a substitute if the selected address was ineligible for the survey, for example, if it was empty when the interviewer called or was no longer PSL accommodation. Interviewers who found more than one household at an address, selected two of them at random.

Interviewers identified all adults aged 16 to 64 in the resident household and selected one of them for interview using the Kish grid method.[4] *(Figure 3.2)*

Nightshelters and day centres

Sampling frames of nightshelters and day centres which met the survey definitions were compiled using information from local authority housing departments, known local lists and by snowballing. This process involved contacting the 26 regional Housing Advice Centres run by Shelter to identify nightshelters and day centres which in turn were contacted to identify others. We then wrote to all these establishments to clarify whether they were eligible for the survey.

A night shelter was eligible if it offered direct access accommodation to people who were homeless and did not have enough money to find alternatives.[5] A day centre was eligible if it offered a daytime meeting place, perhaps with other services, which were targeted specifically at homeless people and if there were people who slept rough amongst their clientele.

If the establishments were eligible, the administrators were asked to keep a one-week diary recording the number of guests who attended each day and met the following criteria for inclusion in the survey:

In nightshelters: aged 16 to 64 years

In day centres: aged 16 to 64 years and slept rough on any one of the past seven nights

Thus it was possible to produce sampling frames of eligible nightshelters and day centres, stratified into broad size bands. It was not cost-effective to include very small establishments; nightshelters and day centres which catered for fewer than 5 eligible adults on average per day were excluded from the sampling frame.

i) Nightshelters

Nightshelters on the sampling frame were stratified by size and 31 were selected: all those with an estimated daily average of 10 or more eligible guests were selected and a subsample of one in two smaller nightshelters was drawn. The remaining six were entered into a pool of reserves to be allocated as substitutes for nightshelters which were found to be ineligible or refused to take part.

For each nightshelter interviewers were given a sampling fraction and a random start. Also a weekday was selected at random and assigned to each nightshelter, indicating on which day of the week all the sampling and almost all the interviewing must take place.

It was necessary for interviewers to ask screening questions of every nightshelter guest to establish whether they were eligible for the

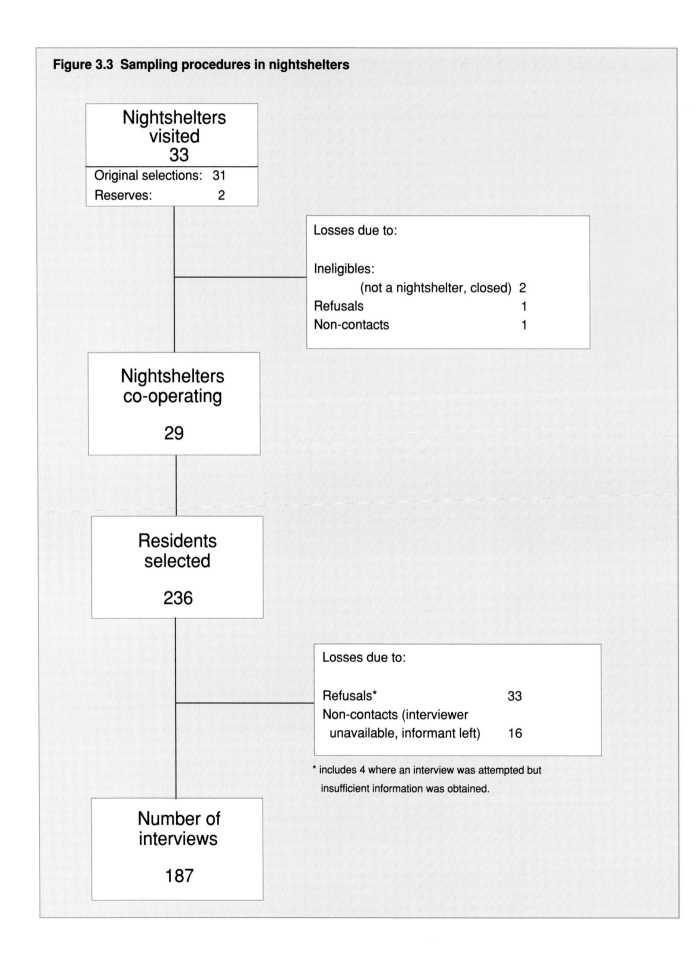

Figure 3.3 Sampling procedures in nightshelters

Nightshelters visited
33
Original selections: 31
Reserves: 2

Losses due to:

Ineligibles:
(not a nightshelter, closed) 2
Refusals 1
Non-contacts 1

Nightshelters co-operating
29

Residents selected
236

Losses due to:

Refusals* 33
Non-contacts (interviewer
unavailable, informant left) 16

* includes 4 where an interview was attempted but
insufficient information was obtained.

Number of interviews
187

Figure 3.4 Sampling procedures in day centres

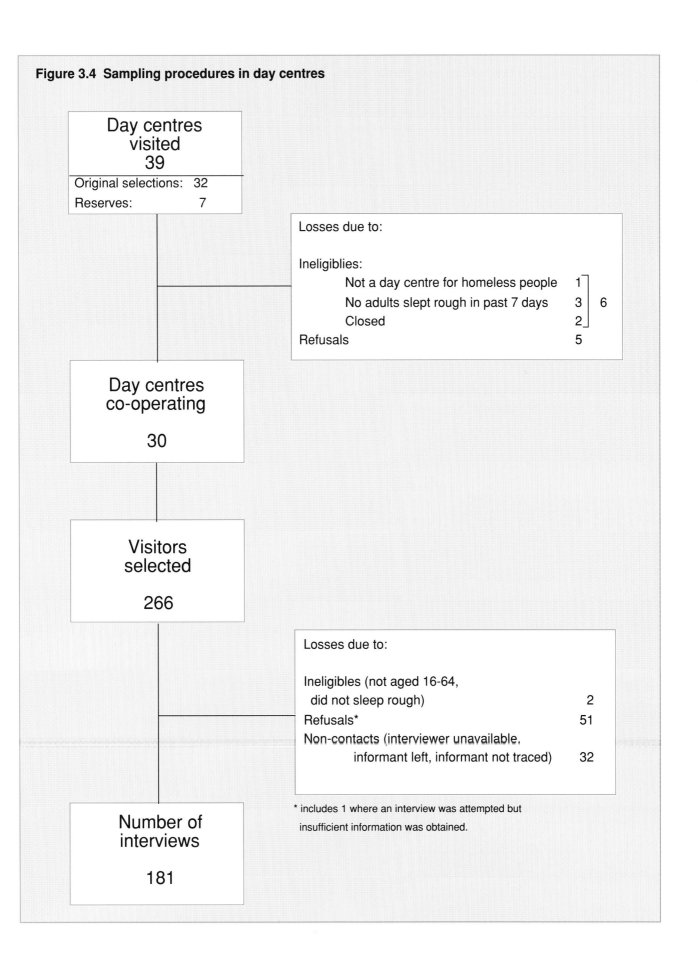

survey, that is whether they were aged 16 to 64 and had not been interviewed previously. Interviewers applied a systematic sampling fraction to those who were eligible and 236 adults were selected for interview. *(Figure 3.3)*

The number of interviewers sent to each nightshelter was kept to a minimum to reduce disruption to staff and residents. Nevertheless, all sampling was scheduled to be conducted on a specified evening and, despite the very limited time available, the majority of interviewing was planned to be completed by the following morning. Furthermore, it could not be guaranteed that the expected number of eligible adults would attend the nightshelter on that night. To ensure that sufficient interviews were obtained in these circumstances, the sampling fractions were set deliberately high (in many establishments, every eligible adult was selected) and there was a possibility that not all selected adults would be interviewed because of interviewer unavailability.

ii) Day centres

Day centres on the sampling frame were stratified by size and 32 were selected: all those with an estimated daily average of 40 or more eligible guests were selected and a subsample of one in two smaller day centres was drawn. The remaining 18 were entered into a pool of reserves to be allocated as substitutes for day centres which were found to be ineligible or refused to take part.

As in nightshelters, each day centre was assigned a sampling fraction and random start, and also a weekday on which all the sampling and the majority of interviewing was to take place.

Interviewers attempted to screen every visitor to the day centre for eligibility by asking a series of questions to ascertain that they were aged 16 to 64, had not previously been interviewed and had slept rough on one of the past seven nights. They then applied a systematic sampling fraction to those who were

eligible and 266 adults were selected for interview. *(Figure 3.4)*

It was planned that all sampling and the majority of interviewing would take place on the sampling day but there was no certainty that the expected number of eligible people would attend the centre that day. Just as in nightshelters, the sampling fraction was kept high and it was acknowledged that sometimes a relatively high number of selected visitors might not be contacted in the time allotted for interviewing.

3.3   Organisation of the interview

The interviewing procedures in hostels and PSL accommodation were similar to those used in the survey in private households.[6] These procedures were modified for nightshelters and day centres, so that the interview was approximately half the length of that in hostels and PSLA.

The first step in hostels, nightshelters and day centres was to conduct a short interview using the Establishments schedule (I) with the administrator or another member of staff. This covered the type of establishment, its client group, funding and the types of facilities provided including health services.

Hostels and PSL accommodation

Every sampled adult was asked Schedule A which covered:

- Socio-demographic characteristics
- Housing circumstances and history
- General health questions including long-standing illness
- Clinical Interview Schedule - Revised (CIS-R) [7]
- The Psychosis Screening Questionnaire (PSQ)[8] and associated questions which indicate the possibility of psychotic disorder

All adults were also given the GHQ12[9] (Schedule GH), for self completion.

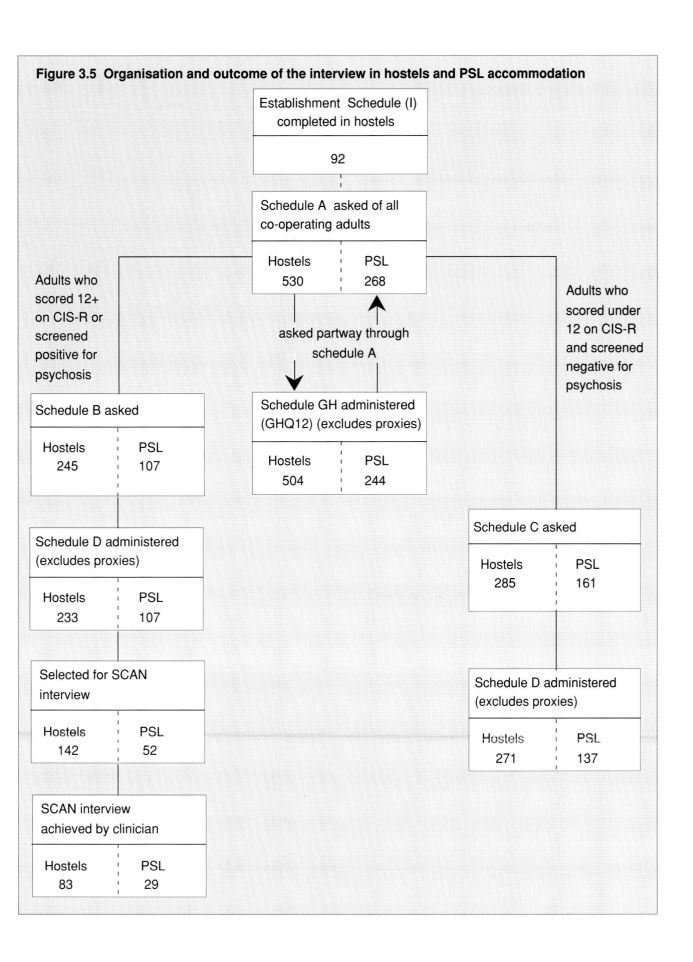

Figure 3.5 Organisation and outcome of the interview in hostels and PSL accommodation

Interviewers were instructed on the importance of obtaining information required for an assessment of mental health as a matter of priority over other survey information as it was anticipated that some interviews might not be completed. They were also allowed to change the question order if they considered it would make the interview more acceptable to the informant. It was therefore recommended that the GHQ12 should be administered early on in the interview, after the general health questions but before the Psychosis Screening Questionnaire.

From their answers to Schedule A, individuals who were at or above the threshold on the CIS-R (a score of 12 or more), and those who gave indications of having a psychotic illness were asked Schedule B which was made up of the following sections:

- Medication and treatment
- Health, social and voluntary care services
- Recent stressful life events
- Social activities and social networks
- Education and employment
- Finances
- Smoking
- Alcohol consumption

Those below the threshold were asked Schedule C, an abridged version of Schedule B, in order to get comparable information. Because these informants were assumed to have no mental health problems, the questionnaire was shortened by omitting the sections on medication and treatment, and use of services.

Finally, all subjects were given a second self-completion questionnaire (Schedule D) covering alcohol dependency among those who drank at least 5 units of alcohol a day on a monthly basis, and drug-taking and the regularity of drug use.

Subjects who could have a psychotic illness were selected for a follow-up clinical interview using SCAN[10] which would be conducted

within a few weeks by a registrar or senior registrar in psychiatry.

The flowchart in Figure 3.5 depicts the organisation of the interview and the path taken by informants in hostels and PSL accommodation through the different interview schedules.

Nightshelters and day centres

There was often only limited time available for interviewing adults in nightshelters and day centres and pilot work showed many informants had difficulty with a long, detailed interview. Hence the interview in nightshelters and day centres was a shortened form of that in hostels and PSL accommodation.

Every sampled adult was asked Schedule DN which covered:

- Socio-demographic characteristics
- Housing circumstances and history
- General health questions including long-standing illness
- The Psychosis Screening Questionnaire (PSQ) and associated questions which indicate the possibility of psychotic disorder
- Medication and treatment
- Health, social and voluntary care services
- Recent stressful life events
- Education and employment
- Finances
- Smoking
- Alcohol consumption

It should be noted that the revised Clinical Interview Schedule (CIS-R) was not asked of these samples; piloting showed it was too lengthy and a significant proportion of informants with poor concentration or with difficulty in recalling events in the previous week were not capable of answering it. Unlike the interview in hostels and PSL accommodation, the routing through the questionnaires was not determined by the outcome of screening questions for neurosis or

Figure 3.6 Organisation and outcome of the interview in nightshelters and day centres

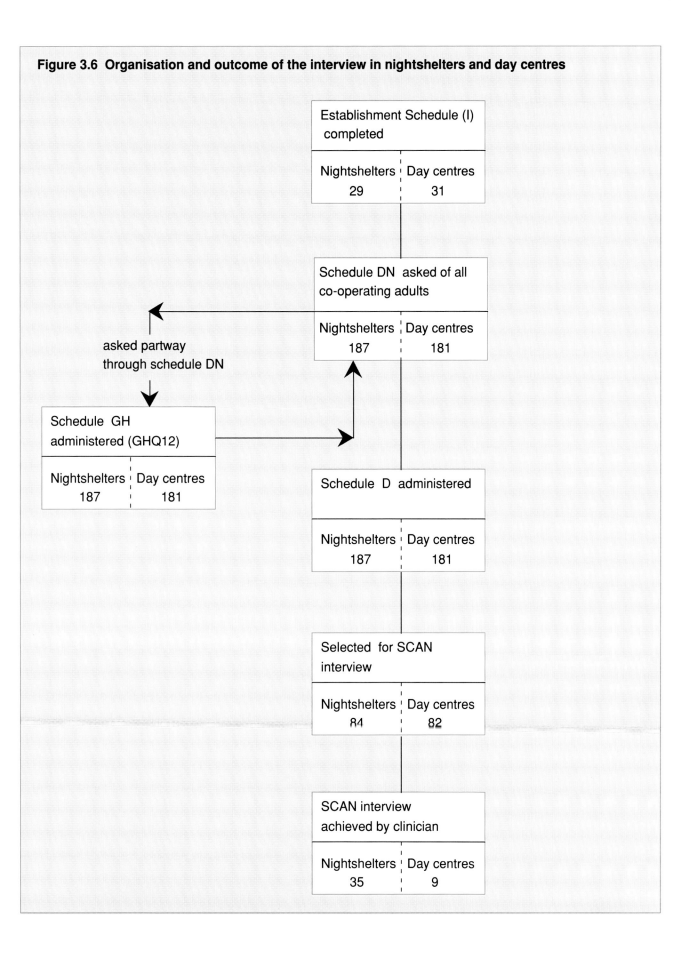

psychosis: all informants were given the same interview. Questions were not asked on social networks and many of the sections covered were less detailed than in hostels and PSL accommodation.

As in hostels and PSL accommodation, all informants were given two self-completion questionnaires:

- Schedule GH, the GHQ12 - again, it was recommended that this should be administered early on in the interview, after the general health questions but before the Psychosis Screening Questionnaire.

- Schedule D, administered at the end of the interview, covering alcohol dependency among those who drank at least 5 units of alcohol a day on a monthly basis, and drug-taking and the regularity of drug use.

Similarly, subjects who were found by the OPCS interviewer possibly to be suffering from a psychotic illness were selected for a follow-up clinical interview by a registrar or senior registrar in psychiatry. Because of difficulties in retracing some informants, particularly in day centres, it was necessary for psychiatrists to attempt a follow-up interview within days of the first interview.

The organisation of the interview in nightshelters and day centres and the path informants took through the interview schedules is shown diagrammatically in Figure 3.6.

3.4   Interviewing procedures

Pre-pilot and pilot surveys

Before carrying out the main stage survey of psychiatric morbidity among homeless people, a pre-pilot and pilot survey were carried out. The pilot survey involved 40 interviews in 14 establishments. The purpose of piloting was to investigate the feasibility of sampling and interviewing among homeless people in the various settings and to develop effective procedures. It was also used to examine and refine questions and the question order which had been successfully used in the surveys in private households and in institutions for mentally ill people, as well as to test the acceptability of the survey among administrators, staff and residents or visitors.

Organisation and training of interviewers

All the interviewers on this survey had previously worked on the survey in private households and were personally briefed on sampling and interviewing procedures for this survey. Interviewers worked in teams in nightshelters and day centres, and also in hostels which had a fast turnover of residents. A team leader was responsible for contacting the administrators and making arrangements for sampling and interviewing.

Maximising response

In order to maximise co-operation, letters were sent to sampled establishments and PSLA addresses explaining the purpose of the survey and that an interviewer would call. Booklets were prepared for administrators and staff in these establishments which detailed how the sampling would be carried out and what the interview would entail. Interviewers made several calls at PSLA addresses and hostels to make contact with selected informants.

Staff help was vital to the success of the survey in hostels, nightshelters and day centres. They were instrumental in explaining the survey to residents and visitors, assisted in drawing up a list of residents in hostels, and helped to arrange appointments to interview selected informants.

The organisation of follow-up interviews to be conducted by clinicians was particularly difficult in day centres and to a lesser extent in nightshelters and hostels because of the difficulty in retracing informants. In order to maximise the chances of making contact with an informant, clinicians were able to telephone staff and check if the informant was present or if an appointment could be made. Despite this, very few SCAN interviews were achieved in day centres. There were three reasons for this. First, many day centre visitors attended irregularly or infrequently, or only stayed for a short amount of time, making re-contact highly unlikely. Second, in large day centres it was difficult for staff to help in identifying a particular informant. Also, clinicians were not available full-time during the hours day centres were open. As was described in Section 2.2, a diagnosis of psychosis was still possible in cases where the SCAN follow-up interview was not achieved.

Introducing the survey

Interviewers were briefed on how to introduce the survey to administrators and staff as well as residents or guests. They were told to avoid using terms such as "psychiatric morbidity" or "mental illness". The results from our pilot surveys indicated that most people could relate to the expressions "health and well-being" and "coping with the stresses and strains of everyday life". The main points covered in the introduction were:

(a)   who the survey was for
(b)   what the survey was about
(c)   why the survey had been extended to include people with housing needs
(d)   how the results would be used
(e)   how their address/establishment was sampled

Proxy information

In some circumstances proxy information was collected, rather than lose information about the selected informant. This was especially relevant when the subject could not answer questions due to a mental health or alcohol-related problem, but also applied to informants who were too physically ill, had a speech or hearing problem, or had language problems.

However, proxy interviews were only carried out where it was felt that the proxy informant knew the selected adult well enough. In hostels, proxy information was only taken from members of the informant's family or staff and not from other residents, and in PSL accommodation it was taken from a member of the informant's family. No proxy information was taken in nightshelters and day centres.

Notes and references

1.   DoE, December 1993 *Information Bulletin 849: Households found accommodation under the homelessness provisions of the 1985 Housing Act: England, Statistics for the third quarter of 1993*, Tables 4b and 5, and Supplementary Table

2.   Scottish Office, Number of households in temporary accommodation at 30 June 1993 (unpublished)

3.   Welsh Office, Number of households accommodated in temporary accommodation at 30 September 1993 (unpublished)

4.   Kish, L., (1965) *Survey Sampling*, J Wiley & Sons Ltd, London

5.   The definition of a nightshelter was based on the definition used for the London Hostels Directory: Resource Information Service (1993) London Hostels Directory, London

6.   The private household survey involved interviews with 10,000 randomly sampled adults in Great Britain.

7.   Lewis, G. and Pelosi, A.J., *Manual of the Revised Clinical Interview Schedule, (CIS-R)*, June 1990, Institute of Psychiatry. See also Lewis, G., Pelosi, A.J., Araya, R.C. and Dunn, G., (1992) Measuring psychiatric disorder in the community: a standardized assessment for use by lay interviewers, *Psychological Medicine*, **22**, 465-486.

8.   Bebbington, P.E., and Nayani, T (1995) 'The Psychosis Screening Questionnaire' *International Journal of Methods in Psychiatric Research*, **5**:11-19

9.   Goldberg, D. and Williams, PA., (1988) *User's Guide to the General Health Questionnaire*, NFER-NELSON

10. *Schedules for Clinical Assessment in Neuropsychiatry*, 1992, WHO, Division of Mental Health, Geneva

4   Characteristics of the sample

4.1   Introduction

This chapter is divided into four sections. Each section is devoted to a description of the socio-demographic characteristics of one of the four samples of homeless people: residents of hostels, adults living in private sector leased accommodation, those staying at nightshelters and people sleeping rough using day centres.

The sections on day centres, nightshelters and hostels also include a brief profile of these institutions, for example, what proportion of hostel residents were living in hostels which were run by local authorities, or were staffed day or night.

4.2   Hostels

Age, sex, ethnicity, marital status, and family unit type

A third of all 530 hostel residents were aged 16 to 24, just over a quarter were aged 25 to 34 and about an eighth were in each of the three other age categories: 35-44, 45-54 and 55-64.

Overall, 70% of hostel residents interviewed for the survey were men and 30% were women. Men and women were equally represented among the 16-24 year olds. The proportion of men rose to 78% of the 25-34 year olds and to 85% of those aged 35 or above.

A quarter of all hostel residents belonged to an ethnic minority, most of them were Black African (10%), Black Caribbean (5%) or did not ascribe themselves to any of the eight ethnic groups developed for the 1991 Census (7%). The representation of ethnic minorities decreased from a third of hostel residents aged 16 to 34 to a fifth of those aged 35 to 44 to just a few percent of those aged 45 and above.

Two thirds of the sample were single and as would be expected this proportion decreased with age from 88% of the 16-24 year olds to 31% of the 45-54 year olds. Sixty per cent of this latter group were either divorced (44%) or separated (16%).

Eight out of ten hostel residents did not live with a family member. Of the twenty two percent of adults interviewed in hostels who were part of homeless families, 9% were lone parents living with their children. *(Table 4.1)*

Education and employment characteristics

About half the sample of hostel residents had no educational qualifications, ranging from 39% of the 16-24 year olds to 68% of the 55-64 year olds. The most well qualified residents were aged 25-44: 25% of the 25-34 year olds and 29% of the 35-44 year olds had at least 'A' level qualifications.

Only 13% of hostel residents were working - 10% full time and 3% part time. Overall, just over a third, 37%, were unemployed and seeking work and a half were economically inactive. The proportion of economically inactive adults aged 55-64 was twice that of the 16-24 year olds: 84% compared with 42%.

The classification of social class was based on the resident's present occupation or last job if presently unemployed. The previous job of the presently unemployed may have been quite a while ago, especially for elderly hostel residents. Nevertheless, one notable finding from analysis by social class is that around a quarter of hostel residents aged 16-24 had never worked . *(Table 4.2)*

Accommodation characteristics

Among the hostel dwellers 71% had their own room. Those who did share rooms were more likely to be the younger residents sharing with one or two others. Most families tended to have just one bedroom.

Overall, about a half of the sample of hostel residents had been in their present accommodation for less than 6 months. However, length of stay was strongly associated with age. For example, 70% of 16-24 year olds had been resident at their present hostel for less than 6 months compared with 50% of 35-44 year olds and 21% of the 55-64 year olds. Although not shown in the tables, no family had been living in a hostel for more than 2 years.

The expectation of moving on to more permanent accommodation was also related to age in that three-quarters of the youngest age group expected to move in the next six months compared with around a half of 25-54 year olds and about a fifth of those aged 55 or above. *(Table 4.3)*

Hostel characteristics

The five hundred and thirty residents who agreed to take part in the survey were living in ninety two hostels. About half the residents were living in hostels run solely by local authorities or in combination with other organisations. The other half were in hostels administered by voluntary or charitable organisations again either by themselves or in combination with other agencies. Overall, 33% of residents were living in hostels which solely had a direct access policy. A slightly higher proportion were staying in hostels where entry was solely by referral. The remaining 23% of hostel dwellers were in places which adopted both means of access. The youngest group of residents, aged 16-24, were far more likely to be living in hostels that had a policy of referral as a means of entry. *(Table 4.4)*

Hostels which cater for homeless people vary considerably in terms of their size, their function, the skill mix of staff, the degree of support they offer to residents and their target group. In the London Hostels Directory[1] combinations of these characteristics have been used to develop a typology of hostels.

Short stay hostel

Accommodation for homeless people for a few weeks or months. Short stay hostels will accept people with no money although they may need to be eligible for benefits or wages

Low support hostel

A low support hostel is for people in housing need but provides only limited support. In many cases they are staffed only by resident wardens with some catering or maintenance support. Many of these hostels are quite large with a large proportion of single rooms.

Semi-supportive hostel

This is accommodation for people living fairly independently with some practical or personal support available. There is daytime but not usually twenty four hour staff. Emphasis is on finding permanent housing and practical preparation for independent living.

Supportive hostel

Accommodation for between six to nine months and a few years. There is a strong emphasis on counselling, education and training to prepare for independent living. There is 24 hour staff cover.

Housing scheme

Organisation running a number of flats, bedsits or shared houses and offering little more support than sensitive management, for example, helping to organise benefit claims. There is a good chance of permanent housing.

Supportive group house

House offering a community atmosphere and other support services. Great importance is put on finding the right people for the right houses through a long assessment process.

Traditional hostel

Large hostel established for many years and traditionally used by people who have been homeless for some time. Many have dormitory or cubicle accommodation but very few single rooms.

Table 4.4 shows that just over three quarters of residents interviewed in the survey were staying in four main types of hostel: supportive (29%), semi-supportive (21%), short-stay (15%) and traditional (12%). One in ten residents were in hostels not covered by the typology; they were staying in probation or bail hostels or single parent refuges. The proportions of residents in supportive and semi-supportive hostels did not vary considerably with age. Whereas younger residents were more likely to be in short-stay hostels, older residents had a greater representation in traditional and low-support hostels.

Homeless people tend to have many problems directly or indirectly associated with their housing difficulties and hostels differ in the extent to which they target people with these difficulties. Many homeless adults were living in hostels which cater for people with a whole range of problems. Table 4.5 shows that between forty and fifty percent of residents were in hostels which targeted young people or those who were unemployed or had alcohol or drug problems or were ex-offenders. Although 36% of hostel dwellers were in places which catered for people with mental health problems, hardly any had beds which were specifically put aside for people with mental health problems.

The youngest group of hostel residents, those aged 16-24, tended to be in hostels which mainly catered for their age group: homeless single people, lone parents or those who have recently left care. In contrast, older hostel residents tended to be in hostels which catered for homeless people with a whole range of problems. For example, among the 55-64 year olds, 90% were in hostels targeting people with alcohol problems, 81% were in hostels looking after ex-offenders and 78% were in accommodation which catered for those with drug problems.

Ninety five percent of hostel residents had staff on their premises which includes 83% who had staff on duty day and night.

A whole range of services were available to hostel residents; some were hostel-based whilst others were brought in when required. The most extensively provided service was giving advice to residents: 9 out of 10 hostel residents were in places which gave advice on housing or resettlement. 84% of residents had the possibility of getting advice on how to live independently and 67% were in hostels providing advice on finding employment. On a more basic level, about two thirds of residents had the opportunity of making or buying meals or snacks at their hostels. The extent of the availability of health services to residents varied by type of service. 59% of the sample were living in hostels that had key workers and 44% had the possibility of contact with a drugs or alcohol counsellor. GPs were available to just over a third of hostel residents. *(Table 4.5)*

Older residents were more likely than younger residents to live in hostels which provided meals or snacks, had drugs or alcohol counselling and access to mental health team services.

Comparison with hostels for people with mental health problems

As part of the OPCS surveys of psychiatric morbidity a sample of residents in institutions which catered for people with mental health problems was also interviewed. This included 125 residents living in hostels designated for this purpose. A comparison of residents from both types of hostel show that homeless hostel residents had a greater proportion of men, those aged 16-34 and unemployed adults. More significantly, a greater proportion of homeless people living in hostels belonged to ethnic minority groups (24% cf 7%) or were married (12% cf 1%). *(Table 4.6)*

4.3   Private sector leased accommodation (PSLA)

Age, sex, ethnicity, marital status, and family unit type

Sixty three percent of homeless adults living temporarily in private sector leased accommodation were women. Just over a third of all residents were aged 16-24, the same proportion were aged 25-34. One of the most striking findings of Table 4.7 is that 44% of the sample belonged to ethnic minorities and this proportion did not vary very much by age. The largest proportion, 48%, was found among the 25-34 year olds. Looking at the distribution of particular ethnic groups by age, 18% of those aged 35 or above were classified as belong to the Asian/Oriental category; three times the proportion of the younger residents.

One of the main differences between homeless people housed temporarily in private sector leased accommodation and those living in or using other premises was that the former group had a greater proportion of couples living with their children. As well as the 49% of respondents living with their partner and children, a further 18% were lone parents, and an additional 16% were young adults living with one or both parents. Only one in nine residents was living in private sector leased accommodation with no other family member. *(Table 4.7)*

Education and employment characteristics

Those living in private sector leased accommodation were similar to hostel residents in their educational attainment. Overall, 43% had no qualifications and the most well qualified group were the 25-34 year olds.

Eighty percent of the sample in private sector leased accommodation were not working and this proportion did not vary considerably by age. The majority, 55%, were economically inactive and the remaining 25% were unemployed. A quarter of all those interviewed had never worked, comprising a third of the 16-24 year olds and a quarter of those aged 35 or over. *(Table 4.8)*

Accommodation characteristics

Two-thirds of the sample had been in their accommodation for less than a year including half who had been there for less than 6 months.

Six in ten residents of private sector leased accommodation expected to leave their present homes in the next 6 months and overall, 4 in 10 expected to move to permanent accommodation. The expectation of a move did not vary much by age yet the youngest group of residents were less likely to know if they were going to move to permanent or other temporary accommodation. *(Table 4.9)*

4.4   Nightshelters

Age, sex, ethnicity and marital status

The personal characteristics of the sample of homeless people using nightshelters presented in Table 4.11 show that 9 in 10 were men, the same proportion were White, and most, 73%, were single. Nearly a quarter, 24%, were divorced or separated. *(Table 4.11)*

Education and employment characteristics

Among those staying in nightshelters, 5 in 10 had no qualifications, 5 in 10 were unemployed, 4 in 10 were economically inactive and 1 in 10 had never worked. Their social class profile was markedly different from those living in hostels and in private sector leased accommodation in that a far smaller proportion of those staying in nightshelters were classified as being in social class I, II, or III Non-manual. *(Table 4.12)*

Accommodation profile

Thirty nine per cent of nightshelter residents had slept rough for at least one night in the seven nights prior to interview including 14% who had spent the previous night sleeping rough. *(Table 4.13)*

When asked about their previous accommodation, 7 out of 8 nightshelter residents said they had stayed in similar accommodation: other nightshelters, bed and breakfast accommodation or hostels. *(Table 4.13)*

Although most of the people using nightshelters had slept rough some time in the past 12 months, about half the sample had spent less than a month doing so.

When asked which was the last place they stayed at which they thought of as home, three quarters stated that this was their own, their parents' or their relatives' accommodation. *(Table 4.14)*

Nightshelter characteristics

Most residents of nightshelters were in places where voluntary and charitable organisations alone or in conjunction with local authorities had the main responsibility.

Between 70-74% of the sample were living in nightshelters which targeted people with mental health problems, or those with alcohol or drug problems, or ex-offenders. Among all nightshelter residents, those aged 16 to 24 rather than those aged 35-64 were living in places which targeted people with a whole range of medical, economic and social problems. *(Table 4.15)*

Practically all residents could get something to eat or drink at their nightshelters and at least 8 in 10 were staying at a place where advice on housing and independent living was provided. As for the provision of health services, about 6 in 10 residents had access to counselling on alcohol and drugs or GP contact and around 5 in 10 had access to mental health services. *(Table 4.15)*

4.5 Adults sleeping rough using day centres

Age, sex, ethnicity and marital status

Nearly 9 in 10 homeless adults who were sleeping rough and used day centres were men. However, their age distribution was slightly different from nightshelter residents: half the sample were aged 35 or over and just 19% overall were aged 16-24. Across all age ranges there were very few day centre users who had a West Indian, African, Asian or Oriental ethnicity. Around two thirds of the sample were single, the remaining third were mainly divorced or separated. *(Table 4.16)*

Education and employment characteristics

About 6 in 10 rough sleepers using day centres had no qualifications and this proportion did not vary significantly with age. Not unexpectedly, fifty percent of rough sleepers were economically inactive and the majority of the other fifty percent were unemployed. Overall the proportion who had never worked was 13% which included 19% of the 16-24 year olds. *(Table 4.17)*

Accommodation profile

All the sample interviewed in day centres had slept rough for at least one night in the past seven nights - that fact as well as their age were the main criteria for inclusion in the survey. About three quarters of the respondents had actually spent the night before they were interviewed on the streets. *(Table 4.18)*

Half the rough sleepers were staying in private accommodation before they became homeless. Overall, 26% were staying with friends or relatives and 14% had their own place. Those aged 16-24 were twice as likely to come from their own or relatives' accommodation than those aged 35 or over: 59% compared with 30%. Conversely, older residents were twice as likely to have stayed previously in hostels, nightshelters, lodgings or B & Bs, than younger residents: 52% compared with 26%. *(Table 4.18)*

When asked about the length of time they had been sleeping rough in the past 12 months, nearly half the sample had reported having spent at least 6 months as rough sleepers with proportions increasing from 37% of the 16-24 year olds to half (51%) of those aged 25 and above. *(Table 4.19)*

When asked which was the last place they stayed at which they thought of as home, three quarters stated that this was their own, their parents' or their relatives' accommodation, exactly the same proportion for residents of nightshelters. That still left 1 in 4 people who thought of an institution as home. *(Table 4.19)*

Day centre characteristics

Most day centre users in the survey were interviewed in day centres which were fully or partly run by voluntary or charitable organisations. Local authorities and direct funding from government provided joint sponsorship.

About 7 in 10 of the sample were using day centres which targeted people with mental health problems, or people with alcohol or drug problems. Whereas half the youngest group of homeless adults, 16 to 24 year olds, attended day centres which specifically catered for people of their age, the older groups went to day centres which catered for a whole range of problems: mental health problems, alcohol and drug problems, being unemployed or an ex-offender. *(Table 4.20)*

Nearly all users of day centres could get tea, a meal or a snack there, which was probably one of the main reasons for their attendance. At least 70% were at day centres where advice was available on housing, independent living or employment. In relation to the availability of health services, between two thirds and three quarters of the sample were interviewed at a day centre which provided mental health services, counselling on alcohol and drugs, or GP contact.

4.6 Comparison of the four homeless samples on some basic characteristics

For all the socio-demographic characteristics used to describe the four homeless samples, those sleeping rough using day centres were similar to residents of nightshelters. The characteristics of hostel residents were more similar to nightshelter residents than tenants of private sector leased accommodation.

More specifically, Figure 4.1 shows that whereas men were mostly found in hostels, nightshelters and day centres, women were more likely to be staying in private sector leased accommodation. These women tended to be different from other homeless adults in that many were part of two-parent or one-parent homeless families rather than single homeless people.

The illustrations in Figure 4.1 also highlight considerable differences between the four samples in terms of age and ethnicity. Just less than 20% of the sample of homeless people sleeping rough who used day centres were aged 16-24 compared with around 30% of residents of hostels and nightshelters and nearly 40% of those in rented accommodation.

In the survey very few people were interviewed in day centres or nightshelters from ethnic minorities, whereas 24% of hostel residents and 44% of those in private sector leased accommodation identified themselves as being from non-White ethnic groups.

The proportions of homeless people who had no qualifications or were economically inactive did not vary very much in each sample.

References

1.   Resource Information Service (1993) London Hostels Directory, London

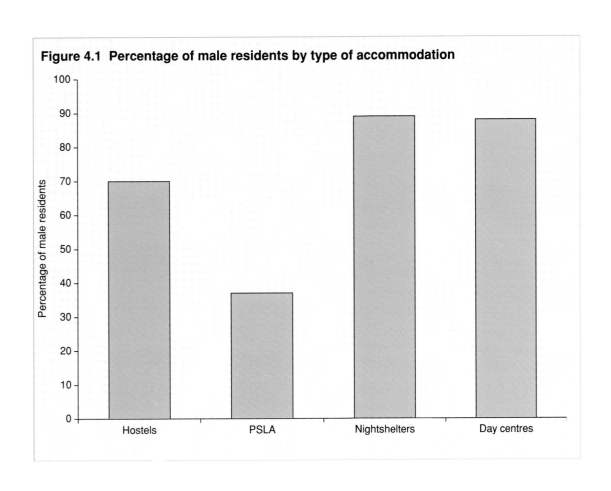

Figure 4.1 Percentage of male residents by type of accommodation

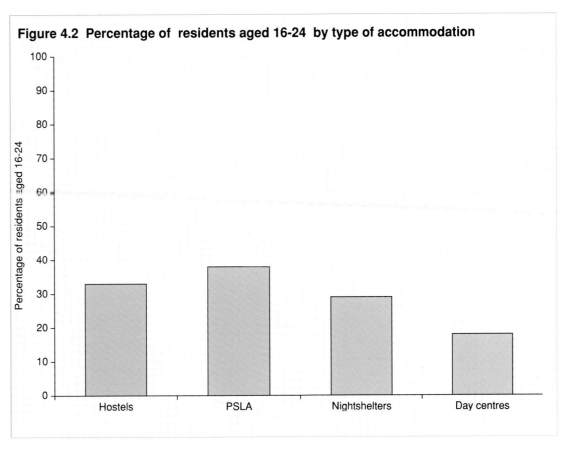

Figure 4.2 Percentage of residents aged 16-24 by type of accommodation

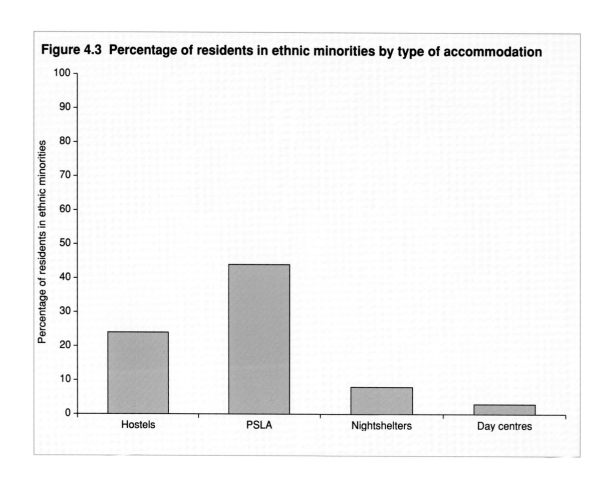

Figure 4.3 Percentage of residents in ethnic minorities by type of accommodation

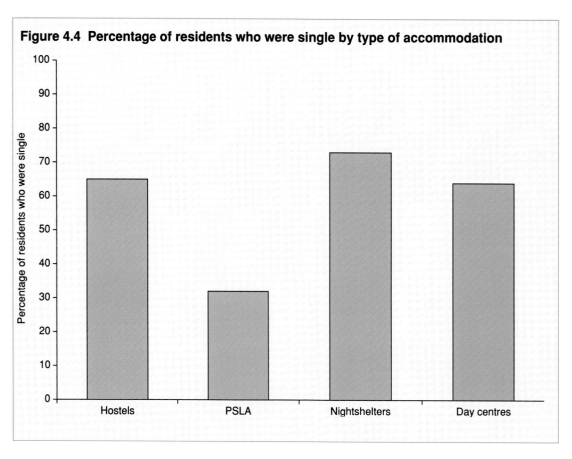

Figure 4.4 Percentage of residents who were single by type of accommodation

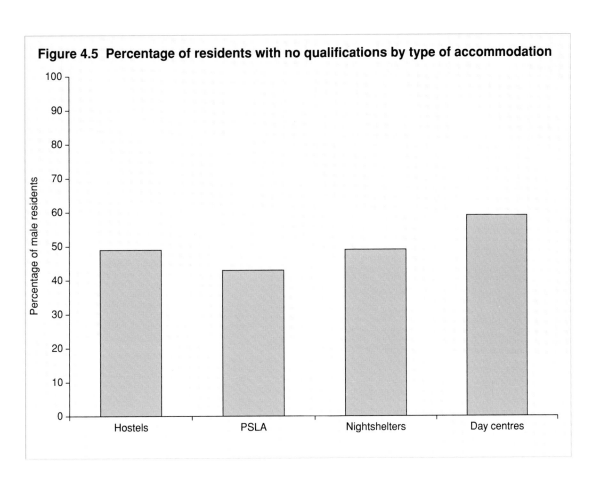

Figure 4.5 Percentage of residents with no qualifications by type of accommodation

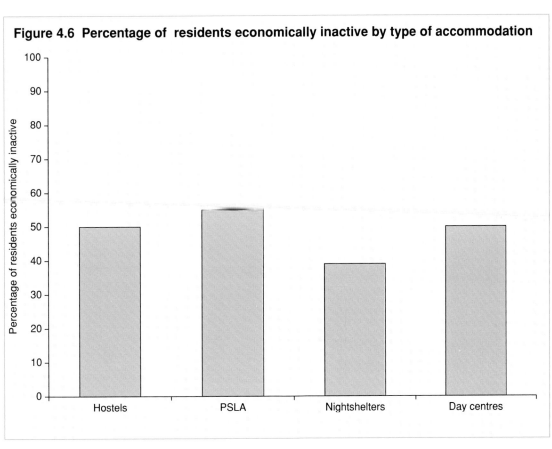

Figure 4.6 Percentage of residents economically inactive by type of accommodation

Table 4.1   Personal characteristics by age

Hostel residents

	Age (grouped)					
	16-24	25-34	35-44	45-54	55-64	All
	%	%	%	%	%	%
Sex						
Men	46	78	84	86	84	70
Women	54	22	16	14	16	30
Ethnicity						
White	67	66	81	100	94	76
West Indian/ African	22	22	7	-	6	15
Asian/ Oriental	1	2	3	0	-	1
Other	10	9	9	-	-	7
Marital status						
Married	1	14	11	7	6	7
Cohabiting	8	9	-	0	-	5
Single	88	68	52	31	46	65
Widowed	-	-	5	3	3	2
Divorced	1	3	20	44	42	15
Separated	2	7	12	16	2	6
Family Unit Type						
Couple, no child(ren)	3	6	6	5	6	5
Couple & child(ren)	6	17	5	2	-	8
Lone parent and child(ren)	20	5	3	-	5	9
One person only	70	72	86	93	89	78
Adult with parents	1	-	-	-	-	0
Adult with one parent	0	-	-	-	-	0
Base	*177*	*146*	*73*	*65*	*70*	*530*
Proportion of hostel residents in each age group	33%	28%	14%	12%	13%	

Table 4.2   Education and employment characteristics by age

Hostel residents

	Age (grouped)					
	16-24	25-34	35-44	45-54	55-64	All
	%	%	%	%	%	%
Qualifications						
A level or higher	13	25	29	11	12	18
GCSE/ O level	35	20	14	10	15	22
Other qualifications	12	9	14	10	5	10
None	39	46	42	68	68	49
Employment status						
Working full time	12	12	9	2	9	10
Working part time	4	5	1	-	-	3
Unemployed	42	44	35	41	7	37
Economically inactive	42	39	55	57	84	50
Social class*						
I	-	3	7	4	-	2
II	6	11	31	7	12	12
III Non-manual	18	13	4	7	4	12
III Manual	15	23	22	28	35	22
IV	23	24	21	36	19	24
V	10	15	12	10	28	14
Armed Forces	1	-	-	-	-	0
Never worked	26	11	2	6	0	13
Not known	0	-	-	2	2	1
Base	*177*	*146*	*73*	*65*	*70*	*530*

*   I = Professional;

II = Employers and managers;

IIINM = Intermediate and Junior Non-Manual;

IIIM = Skilled Manual and own account non professional;

IV = Semi-skilled Manual and Personal service;

V = Unskilled Manual

Table 4.3   Accommodation characteristics by age

Hostel residents

	Age (grouped)					
	16-24	25-34	35-44	45-54	55-64	All
	%	%	%	%	%	%
Accommodation profile						
Lone person in room						
to himself/ herself	58	63	80	89	92	71
Lone person sharing						
with one other	12	8	2	2	-	7
Lone person sharing						
with several others	1	6	4	5	3	4
Living with family						
in one bedroom	25	16	3	4	5	14
Living with family						
in 2+ bedrooms	4	6	11	-	-	5
Length of time in						
present accommodation						
Less than 3 months	49	31	35	12	12	33
3 months < 6 months	21	12	16	19	9	16
6 months < 1 year	21	23	12	20	13	19
1 year < 2 years	8	14	16	17	15	12
2 years < 3 years	2	11	2	17	14	8
3 years or more	-	9	20	15	38	12
Expectation to move in						
next 6 months						
Yes.....						
expect permanent housing	55	36	21	37	17	38
expect temporary housing	5	4	7	4	4	5
not known where	10	14	15	4	-	10
other answers	5	1	3	3	-	3
No or don't know						
if expect to move	25	46	54	52	79	45
Base	*177*	*146*	*73*	*65*	*70*	*530*

Table 4.4   Characteristics of hostels by age of residents

Hostel residents

	Age (grouped)					
	16-24	25-34	35-44	45-54	55-64	All
	%	%	%	%	%	%
Management of hostel*						
Local Authority	55	57	38	64	45	53
Voluntary or charitable organisation	42	48	74	55	52	51
Funded directly from government sources	19	5	14	14	1	12
Private or Housing Associations/ co-ops	4	11	6	7	14	8
DHA/Trust	4	6	2	2	7	4
Other organisation	1	1	4	3	-	1
Access to hostel						
Direct access	19	37	37	35	56	33
Referral	64	41	30	35	19	43
Both means of access	17	22	33	30	26	23
Type of hostel**						
Supportive	31	27	32	33	24	29
Semi-supportive	21	24	24	13	20	21
Short-stay	26	18	6	4	4	15
Traditional	4	9	15	23	20	12
Low support	1	9	10	12	20	8
Housing scheme	2	4	4	2	3	3
Supported group home	-	-	4	4	2	1
Other	14	11	4	9	6	10
Base	*177*	*146*	*73*	*65*	*70*	*530*

*Some hostels were manged by more than one organisation which is why percentages sum to more than 100%

**   Other hostels included: probation hostel, bail hostel, single parent refuge

Table 4.5 Staffing, target group and services offered by age

Hostel residents

	Age (grouped)					
	16-24	25-34	35-44	45-54	55-64	All
	%	%	%	%	%	%
Availability of staff						
Day and night	75	77	88	96	97	83
Daytime only	8	9	9	4	2	7
Few hours a day	10	3	1	-	1	4
Unstaffed	6	11	1	0	-	5
Target group*						
Young homeless	61	41	30	51	47	48
People with alcohol problems	17	41	62	87	90	48
Unemployed people	26	42	54	66	74	46
Ex-offenders	17	41	53	73	81	44
People with drug problems	17	36	56	73	78	43
People with mental health						
problems	16	36	43	63	56	36
People leaving care	29	32	27	48	61	36
Working people	24	26	23	42	47	30
Lone parents	26	18	11	12	6	17
Students	19	17	23	4	19	17
Other groups	57	54	48	31	29	48
Services provided*						
Meals	42	65	84	83	94	66
Tea/snacks	43	63	74	76	78	62
Advice on...						
housing	97	88	85	89	86	90
independent living	94	76	84	82	80	84
jobs	72	66	78	56	56	67
Health services						
key worker	63	47	64	68	62	59
drug/alcohol counsellor	36	37	38	80	54	44
GP	36	34	41	37	32	36
Mental Health Team	26	25	21	59	47	32
other services**	43	28	25	47	29	35
Any other service	19	20	17	33	35	23
Base	*177*	*146*	*73*	*65*	*70*	*530*

*   Hostels provided many services and targeted many different groups which is why
    percentages sum to more than 100%

** Other health workers included: Health visitor, Midwife, Sexual health advisor, OT, CPN,
    Dentist, Optician, Social Worker, Chiropodist

Table 4.6   Comparison of characteristics of two types of hostel resident

	Residents of hostels for homeless people	Residents of hostels for people with mental health problems
	%	%
Sex		
Men	70	59
Women	30	41
Age		
16-24	33	25
25-34	28	29
35-44	14	16
45-54	12	17
55-64	13	13
Ethnicity		
White	76	93
West Indian/ African	15	4
Asian/ Oriental	1	2
Other	7	1
Marital status		
Married/cohabiting	12	1
Single	65	86
Widowed	2	1
Divorced	15	10
Separated	6	1
Qualifications		
A level or higher	18	20
GCSE/O level	22	20
Other qualifications	10	10
None	49	50
Employment status		
Working full time	10	12
Working part time	3	12
Unemployed	37	17
Economically inactive	50	60
Base	*530*	*125*

Table 4.7   Personal characteristics by age

PSLA residents

	Age (grouped)			
	16-24	25-34	35-64	All
	%	%	%	%
Sex				
Men	30	35	49	37
Women	70	65	51	63
Ethnicity				
White	61	52	58	57
West Indian/ African	20	29	15	22
Asian/ Oriental	7	6	18	10
Other	12	13	10	12
Marital status				
Married	18	55	67	45
Cohabiting	13	9	6	10
Single	64	20	6	32
Widowed	-	1	3	1
Divorced	-	7	9	5
Separated	4	9	9	7
Family Unit Type				
Couple, no child(ren)	7	7	3	6
Couple & child(ren)	24	57	70	49
Lone parent and child(ren)	16	21	16	18
One person only	12	10	11	11
Adult with parents	28	-	-	10
Adult with one parent	13	4	-	6
Base	96	98	74	268
Proportion of PSLA residents in each age group	36%	36%	27%	

Table 4.8 Education and employment characteristics by age

PSLA residents

	Age (grouped)			
	16-24	25-34	35-64	All
	%	%	%	%
Qualifications				
A level or higher	18	23	18	20
GCSE/ O level	34	13	9	20
Other qualifications	19	22	8	17
None	28	41	65	43
Employment status				
Working full time	12	14	9	12
Working part time	6	12	6	8
Unemployed	29	14	36	25
Economically inactive	54	60	49	55
Social class*				
I	-	-	-	-
II	4	11	19	11
III Non-manual	29	17	8	19
III Manual	5	24	19	16
IV	22	21	17	20
V	5	13	13	10
Armed Forces	-	-	-	-
Never worked	34	14	24	24
Base	*96*	*98*	*74*	*268*

* I = Professional; II = Employers and managers; IIINM = Intermediate and
Junior Non-Manual; IIIM = Skilled Manual and own account non-professional;
IV = Semi-skilled Manual and Personal service; V = Unskilled Manual

Table 4.9 Accommodation characteristics by age

PSLA residents

	Age (grouped)			
	16-24	25-34	35-64	All
	%	%	%	%
Length of time in present accommodation				
Less than 3 months	34	28	29	30
3 months < 6 months	18	15	29	20
6 months < 1 year	16	25	10	18
1 year < 2 years	17	11	12	14
2 years < 3 years	13	8	13	12
3 years or more	2	12	6	7
Expectation to move in next 6 months				
Yes.....				
expect permanent housing	36	43	45	41
expect temporary housing	4	2	5	4
not known where	22	9	3	12
other answers	-	5	1	2
No or don't know if expect to move	38	40	47	41
Base	*96*	*98*	*74*	*268*

Table 4.10 Comparison of characteristics of PSLA residents with renters from private household survey

	Residents of PSLA from homeless survey	Renters of accommodation from private household survey
	%	%
Sex		
Men	37	47
Women	63	53
Age		
16-24	36	26
25-34	36	28
35-44	18	18
45-54	7	13
55-64	2	14
Ethnicity		
White	57	94
West Indian/ African	22	3
Asian/ Oriental	10	2
Other	12	1
Family unit type		
Couple, no child(ren)	6	18
Couple & child(ren)	49	32
Lone parent & child(ren)	18	13
One person only	11	24
Adult with parents	10	7
Adult with one parent	6	5
Qualifications		
A level or higher	20	22
GCSE/O level	20	23
Other qualifications	17	12
None	43	44
Employment status		
Working full time	12	37
Working part time	8	13
Unemployed	25	16
Economically inactive	55	34
Base	*268*	*2664*

Table 4.11   Personal characteristics by age

Nightshelter residents

	Age (grouped)			
	16-24	25-34	35-64	All
	%	%	%	%
Sex				
Men	82	87	97	89
Women	18	13	3	11
Ethnicity				
White	90	83	99	91
West Indian/ African	9	8	-	5
Asian/ Oriental	-	-	1	-
Other	1	9	-	3
Marital status				
Married	-	2	2	1
Cohabiting	1	1	-	1
Single	95	83	50	73
Widowed	-	-	2	1
Divorced/ separated	4	13	47	24
Base	*54*	*58*	*73*	*185*
Proportion of nightshelter residents in each age group	29%	31%	40%	

Table 4.12   Education and employment characteristics by age

Nightshelter residents

	Age (grouped)			
	16-24	25-34	35-64	All
	%	%	%	%
Qualifications				
A level or higher	10	36	12	19
GCSE/ O level	32	22	18	23
Other qualifications	8	7	11	9
None	50	35	60	49
Employment status				
Working full time	2	1	6	3
Working part time	2	3	5	3
Unemployed	64	49	52	54
Economically inactive	32	48	36	39
Social class*				
I	-	-	-	-
II	1	8	2	3
III Non-manual	17	3	3	7
III Manual	26	18	25	23
IV	29	31	30	30
V	16	24	36	26
Armed Forces	-	5	-	2
Never worked	12	10	5	9
Base	*54*	*58*	*73*	*185*

*   I = Professional; II = Employers and managers; IIINM = Intermediate and
    Junior Non-Manual; IIIM = Skilled Manual and own account non–professional;
    IV = Semi-skilled Manual and Personal service; V = Unskilled Manual

Table 4.13   Accommodation profile by age

Nightshelter residents

	Age (grouped)			
	16-24	25-34	35-64	All
	%	%	%	%
Spent last night sleeping rough	**14**	**21**	**10**	**14**
Slept rough on any of the past 7 nights	**34**	**48**	**35**	**39**
Type of previous accommodation				
Lodgings or hostel				
Nightshelter	85	63	89	80
Bed and breakfast	1	10	2	4
Hostel/ resettlement unit	3	-	6	3
Private accommodation				
Friends or relatives	6	16	2	7
Parents' home	6	5	-	3
Squat	-	5	-	2
Prisons / borstals				
Prison/ remand/ police cell	-	-	1	0
Base	*54*	*58*	*73*	*185*

Table 4.14 Accommodation history by age

Nightshelter residents

	Age (grouped)			
	16-24	25-34	35-64	All
	%	%	%	%
Length of time sleeping rough in past 12 months				
Less than a week*	38	38	36	37
1 week < 1 month	15	10	16	14
1 month < 6 months	17	24	13	17
6 months < 1 year	20	25	22	22
All the time	-	3	-	1
Not known	10	-	14	9
Last place thought of as home				
Private accommodation				
Informant's own accommodation	17	54	48	41
Parents' home	35	16	8	18
Friends or relatives	24	10	14	15
At foster parents	1	-	-	0
Squat	1	-	-	1
Lodgings/ hostel				
Hostel/ resettlememt unit	4	12	4	6
Lodgings	2	-	4	2
Bed and breakfast	1	-	3	2
Nightshelter	1	-	4	2
Homes				
Children's home	6	-	-	2
Old people's home	-	-	1	0
Hospitals/ medical units				
Psychiatric unit/ hospital	3	-	2	2
Alcohol unit	-	-	1	0
Prisons/ Borstals				
Prison/ remand/ police cell	1	4	2	2
Current accommodation	1		9	4
Never had a "home"	1	2	1	1
Base	*54*	*58*	*73*	*185*

* Includes those who did not sleep rough in past 12 months

Table 4.15 Characteristics of nightshelters by age

Nightshelter residents

	Age (grouped)			
	16-24	25-34	35-64	All
	%	%	%	%
Management of nightshelter*				
Voluntary or charitable organisation	88	83	90	88
Local authority	53	47	22	49
DHA/Trust	35	35	7	24
Funded directly from government sources	4	9	14	10
Privately run	4	16	2	7
Target group*				
People with mental health problems	83	82	62	74
People with alcohol problems	83	82	62	74
Ex-offenders	82	80	59	72
People with drug problems	83	78	56	70
Unemployed people	70	77	41	60
People leaving care	75	68	33	55
Young homeless	84	58	28	53
Working people	58	42	24	39
Students	11	23	12	15
Lone parents	9	15	4	9
Other groups	13	38	44	34
Services provided*				
Meals	92	99	100	97
Tea/snacks	92	96	94	94
Advice on...				
housing	93	90	92	92
independent living	85	79	80	81
jobs	68	56	44	55
Health services				
key worker	27	38	33	33
drug/alcohol counsellor	60	69	56	61
GP	55	51	65	58
Mental Health Team	44	46	49	47
other services**	23	32	22	25
Any other service	18	28	10	18
Base	*54*	*58*	*73*	*185*

* Nightshelters provided many services and targeted many different groups which is why
percentages sum to more than 100%

** Other health workers included: Health visitor, Midwife, Sexual health advisor, OT, CPN,
Dentist, Optician, Social Worker

Table 4.16 Personal characteristics by age

Homeless adults sleeping rough using day centres

	Age (grouped)			
	16-24	25-34	35-64	All
	%	%	%	%
Sex				
Men	77	92	89	88
Women	23	8	11	12
Ethnicity				
White	96	97	98	97
West Indian/ African	2	2	1	1
Asian/ Oriental	-	-	0	0
Other	3	2	-	1
Marital status				
Married	2	2	2	2
Cohabiting	3	2	1	2
Single	86	75	49	64
Widowed	2	1	4	3
Divorced/ separated	8	19	44	30
Base	*34*	*57*	*91*	*181*
Proportion of Day centre users in each age group	19%	31%	50%	

Table 4.17 Education and employment characteristics by age

Homeless adults sleeping rough using day centres

	Age (grouped)			
	16-24	25-34	35-64	All
	%	%	%	%
Qualifications				
A level or higher	8	9	18	13
GCSE/ O level	24	19	11	16
Other qualifications	9	7	15	11
None	60	65	55	59
Employment status				
Working full time	6	5	1	3
Working part time	7	7	3	5
Unemployed	60	48	32	42
Economically inactive	26	40	64	50
Social class*				
I	-	-	3	1
II	2	13	6	7
III Non-manual	15	2	5	6
III Manual	30	23	34	30
IV	29	28	17	23
V	6	23	25	21
Armed Forces	-	-	0	0
Never worked	19	11	11	13
Base	*34*	*57*	*91*	*181*

*   I = Professional; II = Employers and managers; IIINM = Intermediate and
      Junior Non-Manual; IIIM = Skilled Manual and own account non-professional;
      IV = Semi-skilled Manual and Personal service; V = Unskilled Manual

Table 4.18   Accommodation profile by age

Homeless adults sleeping rough using day centres

	Age (grouped)			
	16-24	25-34	35-64	All
	%	%	%	%
Spent last night sleeping rough	**67**	**81**	**78**	**77**
Slept rough on any of the past 7 nights	**100**	**100**	**100**	**100**
Type of previous accommodation				
Private accommodation				
Friends or relatives	46	35	14	26
Informant's own accommodation	13	12	16	14
Parents' home	8	7	2	5
Squat	1	2	6	4
Provided with work	-	-	2	1
Lodgings or hostel				
Hostel/ resettlement unit	8	13	28	20
Nightshelter	10	9	14	12
Lodgings	-	10	0	3
Bed and breakfast	8	1	10	7
Hospitals/ medical units				
General hospital	-	-	1	1
Psychiatric unit/ hospital	-	1	-	0
Prisons / borstals				
Prison/ remand/ police cell	-	7	1	3
Young offenders institution	2	-	-	0
Other place	**6**	**4**	**4**	**4**
Not known	**-**	**-**	**2**	**1**
Base	*34*	*57*	*91*	*181*

Table 4.19 Accommodation history by age

Homeless adults sleeping rough using day centres

	Age (grouped)			
	16-24	25-34	35-64	All
	%	%	%	%
Length of time sleeping rough in past 12 months				
Less than a week	14	4	6	7
1 week < 1 month	9	10	10	10
1 month < 6 months	39	34	29	32
6 months < 1 year	35	34	33	33
All the time	2	16	18	14
Not known	-	2	4	3
Last place thought of as home				
Private accommodation				
Informant's own accommodation	24	24	41	33
Parents' home	27	42	15	26
Friends or relatives	18	6	16	13
At foster parents	-	4	-	1
Squat	-	1	-	0
Lodgings/ hostel				
Hostel/ resettlememt unit	5	9	12	10
Lodgings	6	-	2	2
Bed and breakfast	6	2	4	4
Nightshelter	2	1	0	1
Hospitals/ medical units				
Psychiatric unit/ hospital	2	-	-	0
Alcohol unit	-	4	-	1
Prisons/ Borstals				
Prison/ remand/ police cell	1	3	-	1
Other	5	2	3	3
Don't know	-	-	2	1
Current accommodation	2	3	2	2
Never had a "home"	2	-	1	1
Base	*34*	*57*	*91*	*181*

Table 4.20 Characteristics of day centres by age

Homeless adults sleeping rough using day centres

	Age (grouped)			
	16-24	25-34	35-64	All
	%	%	%	%
Management of day centre*				
Voluntary or charitable organisation	86	92	97	94
Local authority	20	41	25	29
Funded directly from government sources	22	27	16	21
DHA/Trust	5	12	8	9
Privately run	11	4	5	6
Target group*				
People with mental health problems	32	82	73	69
People with alcohol problems	32	82	73	69
People with drug problems	32	82	73	69
Ex-offenders	34	60	58	54
People leaving care	19	52	45	43
Unemployed people	24	49	37	39
Working people	12	27	18	20
Young homeless	46	10	15	19
Lone parents	2	17	10	11
Students	12	-	-	2
Other groups	56	73	61	64
Services provided*				
Meals	92	100	97	97
Tea/snacks	100	100	98	99
Advice on...				
housing	100	100	92	96
independent living	89	92	84	88
jobs	86	83	57	71
Health services				
Mental Health Team	56	80	66	71
drug/alcohol counsellor	66	80	66	71
GP	56	68	66	65
key worker	34	37	28	32
other services**	67	85	70	74
Any other service	74	61	51	58
Base	*34*	*57*	*91*	*181*

*   Day centres provided many services and targeted many different groups which is why
      percentages sum to more than 100%

** Other health workers included: Health visitor, Midwife, Sexual health advisor, OT, CPN,
      Dentist, Optician, Social Worker

5 Residents of hostels

Summary

Prevalence of psychiatric morbidity

- Just less than half the residents of hostels suffered from fatigue and sleep problems and a third of the sample had significant symptoms of worry and irritability.

- Thirty eight per cent of residents were on or above the threshold score of 12 on the CIS-R, and 28% overall had very high scores, (18 or over).

- 1 in 7 hostel residents were found to have mixed anxiety and depressive disorder, 1 in 8 had depressive episode, and the same proportion had GAD. One in ten residents had a phobic disorder.

- Half the sample with depressive episode had severe depression and half of those with phobia suffered from agoraphobia.

- The prevalence of psychosis among homeless people living in hostels was found to be 8%.

- Sixteen per cent of hostel residents were defined as alcohol dependent, with 10% overall having severe alcohol dependence.

- Six per cent of hostel residents were assessed as dependent on non-cannabinoid drugs.

Use of alcohol, drugs and tobacco

- Fourteen per cent of hostel residents were very heavy drinkers: 10% of those with no neurotic disorder and 18% among those with a neurotic disorder.

- Fifty seven per cent of those living in hostels were drug users with 34%, overall using cannabis.

- Two-thirds of hostel residents smoked cigarettes.

Long-standing illness, treatment and service use

- Physical illnesses were reported by 41% of residents and mental illnesses by 11%.

- A long-standing mental complaint was self-reported by 20% of those with neurosis and for 6% of those found to have no neurotic disorder.

- Forty per cent of women and 28% of men living in hostels had consulted a GP about a mental complaint in the past year.

- Over half (56%) of hostel residents had some form of secondary care in the past 12 months, while a third just had contact with a GP.

- A third (35%) of hostel residents with a neurotic disorder said they had a key worker.

- Overall, 40% of those with a neurotic disorder were receiving some form of treatment.

Economic, financial and social circumstances

- Twelve per cent of men and 18% of women resident in hostels were working.

- Three quarters of all hostel residents were in receipt of some state benefit;

almost two thirds (64%) were receiving Income Support.

- A quarter (27%) of hostel residents with a neurotic disorder had a primary support group of three or fewer people, compared with 19% of those with no neurotic disorder.

- Half of those with a neurotic disorder, and 37% of those with no disorder did not feel close to anyone who lived at their address.

- Two-thirds of adults with a neurotic disorder and a third of those without a disorder had experienced two or more stressful life events in the past six months.

5.1 Introduction

This chapter consists of three sections. In the first section the prevalence of psychosis, neurotic disorders, alcohol and drug dependence is presented. This is followed by a description of hostel residents in terms of the following characteristics:

- use of alcohol, drugs and tobacco
- self-reports of long-standing physical and mental health problems
- contact with health services and treatment for mental health problems
- economic activity
- social functioning
- experience of recent stressful life events

These characteristics are related to the presence or absence of neurotic disorders.

5.2 Prevalence of psychiatric morbidity

Neurotic symptoms and disorders

The extent of neurotic symptomatology among hostel residents was assessed from their

responses to the revised Clinical Interview Schedule (CIS-R). Ninety four percent of the sample (499 out of 530) managed this part of the interview.

The two most prevalent neurotic symptoms were sleep problems and fatigue, affecting just less than half of the residents, followed by worry and irritability experienced by about a third of the sample. The next most frequently occurring symptoms were depression and depressive ideas, each affecting about 3 in 10 residents. Even the least prevalent neurotic symptoms - panic and worry about physical health - were found among 11% of informants. (*Figure 5.1*)

The distribution of the sum of the scores from all sections of the CIS-R, illustrated in Figure 5.2, shows that 38% of residents were on or above the threshold score of 12, indicative of significant neurotic psychopathology. The corresponding proportion among residents of private households was 14%. The proportion of hostel residents who had very high scores, (18 or over) was four times that found in the private household survey (28% compared with 7%). (*Figure 5.2*)

After applying diagnostic algorithms to the CIS-R data, 1 in 7 hostel residents were found to have mixed anxiety and depressive disorder, 1 in 8 had depressive episode, and the same proportion had Generalised Anxiety Disorder (GAD). One in ten residents had a phobic disorder. The diagnostic algorithms permit the classification of depressive episode by severity and of phobic disorders by type. Half the sample with depressive episode had severe depression and half of those with phobia suffered from agoraphobia. (*Figure 5.3*)

Residents who fulfilled several diagnostic criteria are represented in each group. Thus Figure 5.4 shows that 13% of residents had comorbid neurotic disorders - 10% fulfilling the criteria for 2 neurotic disorders and 3% with 3 or 4 disorders. (*Figures 5.3 and 5.4*)

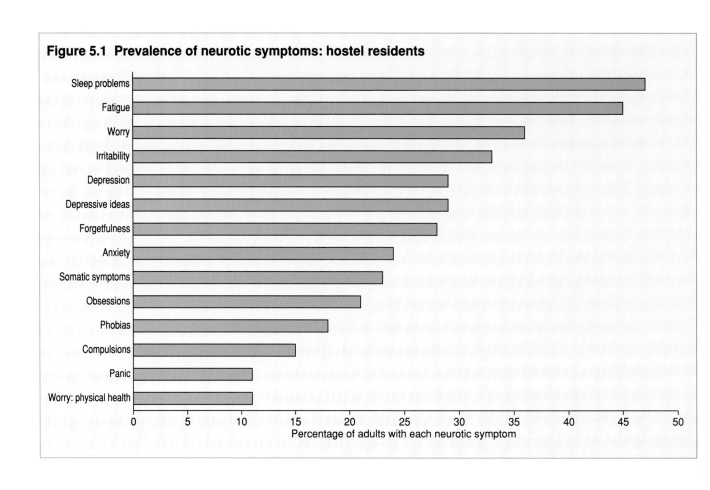

Figure 5.1 Prevalence of neurotic symptoms: hostel residents

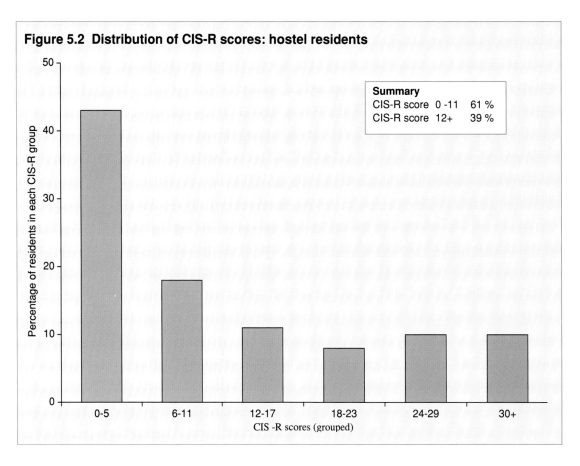

Figure 5.2 Distribution of CIS-R scores: hostel residents

Summary
CIS-R score 0 -11   61 %
CIS-R score 12+   39 %

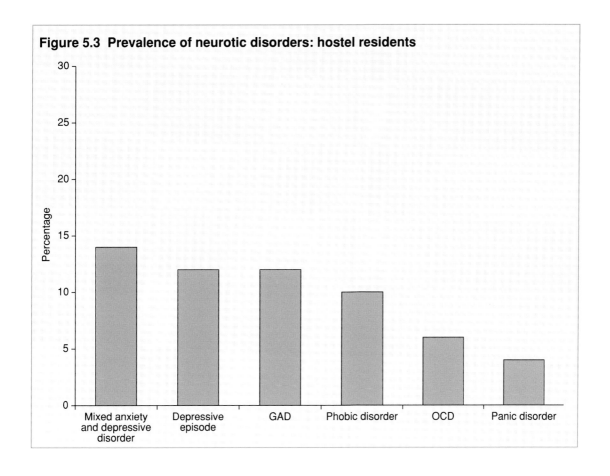

Figure 5.3 Prevalence of neurotic disorders: hostel residents

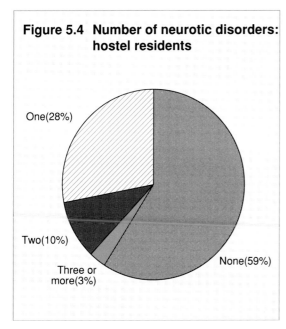

Figure 5.4   Number of neurotic disorders: hostel residents

One(28%)

Two(10%)

Three or more(3%)

None(59%)

Apart from the CIS-R, hostel residents were also administered the GHQ12. Not unexpectedly, the pattern of the distribution of GHQ12 score was similar to that of the CIS-R, with 39% of the sample having a score of 4 or more including 10% with a score of 11 or 12. *(Figure 5.5)*

Psychotic disorders

Chapter 2 of this report gives a detailed account of how psychosis was assessed for all four samples of homeless people. By examining sift criteria (self reports, the use of antipsychotic medication, and the Psychosis Screening Questionnaire), nearly a third of the sample were found to have screened positive for psychosis. However, after taking account of the results of follow up SCAN interviews, and the evaluation by expert psychiatric epidemiologists of descriptive vignettes, the prevalence of psychosis among homeless people living in hostels was found to be 8%. Half of those classified as having psychosis were identified from SCAN interviews. *(Table 5.1)*.

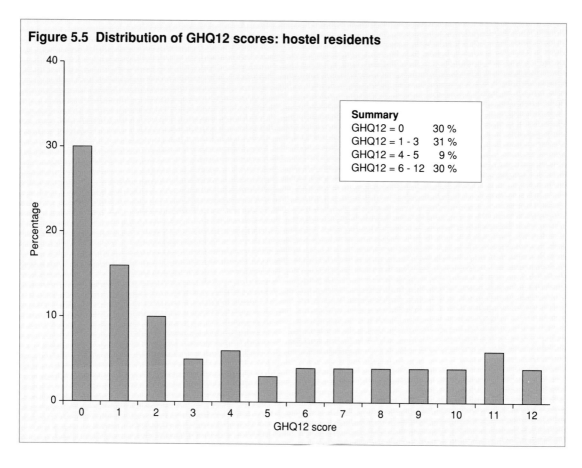

Figure 5.5 Distribution of GHQ12 scores: hostel residents

Summary
GHQ12 = 0   30 %
GHQ12 = 1 - 3   31 %
GHQ12 = 4 - 5   9 %
GHQ12 = 6 - 12   30 %

Co-occurrence of psychiatric disorders

The prevalence of psychosis and each neurotic disorder have so far been examined independently, without the application of any hierarchical rules. In summary 8% of hostel residents had psychosis and 41% had a neurotic disorder. When psychosis is treated as 'trumping' any neurotic disorder, the overall prevalence of neurotic disorders is reduced to 38%. When a hierarchy is imposed on the neurotic disorders the prevalence of depressive episode hardly changes but the proportion of residents with GAD and phobia decreases from 9% to 4% and for OCD from 5% to 2%. *(Table 5.2)*

Alcohol and drug dependence

Sixteen per cent of hostel residents were defined as alcohol dependent, using the private household survey definition. With a more stringent definition, 10% of residents were defined as having severe alcohol dependence. See Appendix B for measures of alcohol and drug dependence. *(Table 5.3)*

Six percent of hostel residents were assessed as non-cannabinoid drug dependent; 3% were solely dependent on non-cannabinoids - hypnotics, stimulants and hallucinogens, while the remaining 3% were also categorised as cannabis dependent (on the loose criteria of regular use which is likely to be over-inclusive). A further 5% of respondents were categorised as cannabis dependent only. About 1 in 5 of those with drug dependence were also alcohol dependent (data not shown in table). *(Table 5.4)*

5.3 Socio-demographic characteristics by type of disorder

There were some quite noticeable differences in the socio-demographic characteristics of hostel residents according to whether they were assessed as having psychosis, a neurotic disorder, severe alcohol dependence or drug dependence. Although these four diagnostic categories are not mutually exclusive, Table 5.5 still shows some marked differences between these groups:

- Eighty six per cent of adults with drug dependence were men and overall 57% were aged 16-24, the largest proportions across all diagnostic groups.

- Although 7% of all hostel residents were married, none of those with psychosis, alcohol or drug dependence were married.

- Nearly all residents, with psychosis, alcohol or severe drug dependence, 95%, were living alone compared with 77% of the group with a neurotic disorder.

- About 7 in 10 residents with alcohol dependence had no educational qualifications compared with 6 in 10 of those with psychosis or drug dependence, and 5 in 10 of the group with neuroses.

- Three quarters of those with psychosis were economically inactive, compared with a half of hostel residents with either alcohol dependence or neurosis. Although, overall, 94% of the drug dependent group were not working, 58% were seeking work and 36% were economically inactive.

The following sections (5.4-5.9) present data on a range of topics for hostel residents with and without a neurotic disorder as measured by the CIS-R; those with a psychotic disorder are excluded from analysis throughout these sections, due to the very different nature of their mental illness. There were insufficient cases to allow analysis of those with psychotic disorders as a separate group.

5.4 Use of alcohol, drugs and tobacco

Use of alcohol

This section reports on current drinking status and reasons for stopping drinking alcohol. It then looks at the amount of alcohol people were consuming, and at symptoms of alcohol dependence.

A quarter of adults living in hostels (24%) were categorised as non-drinkers at the time of interview. While 10% had always been non-drinkers, 14% were ex-drinkers; over half of these ex-drinkers reported that health reasons had led them to stop drinking alcohol (data not shown). While drinking status did not vary according to the presence or absence of a neurotic disorder, among ex-drinkers, health reasons were more prominent as a reason for stopping drinking among those with a neurotic disorder compared with those without such a disorder. *(Table 5.6)*

Twenty two per cent of hostel residents were drinking more than the recommended sensible level; this is identical to the proportion found among adults in private households. However, very heavy drinkers represented 14% of hostel residents, compared with only 5% of those in private households. While 10% of those with no neurotic disorder were very heavy drinkers, the proportion rose to 18% among those with a neurotic disorder. Not surprisingly, alcohol dependence is closely related to consumption, with the heaviest drinkers most likely to be alcohol dependent (data not shown). Severe alcohol dependence was recorded for 13% of those with a neurotic disorder compared with 7% of those without. Alcohol dependence was assessed according to the experience of various symptoms of dependence; symptomatic behaviour was significant for 24% of hostel residents with and 12% without a neurotic disorder, loss of control for 18% and 8% respectively and binge drinking for 9% and 7%. *(Tables 5.7, 5.8 and 5.9)*

Use of drugs

This section presents data both on the use of illicit drugs, and about dependence on these drugs among hostel residents. Compared with adults in the private household survey, drug use was far more widespread among this population. Young men were most likely to report using drugs, 57% of those in hostels were users of any drug compared with 19% of men aged 16-24 in the private household survey. A third of women in hostels in the youngest age cohort used drugs compared with a tenth of those in the private household survey.*(Table 5.10)*

Use of all types of drugs was more prevalent among hostel residents with a neurotic disorder compared with those having no such disorder; cannabis was used by twice the proportion in the former group (34% compared with 16%) while hallucinogens and opiates were used by four times as many of those with neurotic disorders. Compared with adults with no neurotic disorder, the private household survey also found higher prevalence of drug use among adults with a neurotic disorder, however drug use was even more prevalent among hostel residents with no neurotic disorder than among adults in private households with a neurotic disorder. *(Table 5.11)*

Non-cannabinoid drug dependence was recorded for 10% of those with a neurotic disorder, and for 4% of hostel residents with no neurotic disorder; 5% and 1% respectively were dependent on opiates, mostly heroin. *(Table 5.12)*

Eight per cent of hostel residents admitted that they had injected themselves with drugs; 2% had shared injection equipment. In the past month, 2% had injected drugs and 1% had shared equipment (data not shown).

Use of tobacco

Cigarette smoking was about twice as prevalent among hostel residents compared with the private household population; 67% of hostel residents currently smoked compared with 32% of those in private households. In contrast to the private household population, among hostel residents, there was little variation in smoking behaviour according to the presence or absence of a neurotic disorder. *(Table 5.13)*

5.5 Self-reported illness

Survey respondents were asked whether they had any long-standing illnesses. Physical illnesses were reported by 41% and mental illnesses by 11%. A long-standing physical illness was reported by half of those with a neurotic disorder, compared with a third of those with no neurotic disorder; these proportions are almost identical to those found in the private household population. A long-standing mental complaint was self-reported by 20% of those who had a neurotic disorder, and by 6% of those found to have no neurotic disorder. *(Table 5.14)*

The most common physical complaints were musculo-skeletal and respiratory system complaints. Respiratory, nervous system and eye complaints were notably more prevalent among the hostel population than among those in private households; although differences were not massive, it should be remembered that the hostel population was younger on average than the general population, and these disorders are increasingly prevalent with age. *(Table 5.15)*

5.6 Use of services and treatment

GPs

The survey examined the ease of access to medical treatment among homeless people. Over 90% of hostel residents with and without a neurotic disorder knew of a doctor or medical centre they could go to if necessary. Over 90% were registered with a doctor, however it is important to remember that the doctor they were registered with was not necessarily the same as the one they would visit under their present circumstances. GP consultations were in fact higher among hostel residents than those in private households, both in the past 2 weeks, and in the past 12 months. Those in hostels were far more likely to have consulted a GP about a mental complaint in the past year - 40% of women and 28% of men had done so, compared with 16% and 8% respectively of those in private households. In both samples the proportion of such consultations was higher among adults with a neurotic disorder, however it is interesting that the overall rates of consultations for a mental complaint among all hostel residents were almost identical to the rates among men and women with neurotic disorders in the private household population. This suggests that homeless people may find it more acceptable to discuss their mental health with a doctor. *(Tables 5.16 & 5.17)*

Hospitals

For adults with a neurotic disorder, information was collected about any contact with services in a hospital over the past 12 months, and about whether hospital stays or visits were for a physical complaint, a mental complaint, or both. Twenty four per cent of hostel residents reported an in-patient stay for a physical health problem and 5% had been hospitalised for a mental problem. Among the private household population 13% and 1% had in-patient stays for physical and mental complaints respectively (none had a stay for both types of complaint). Thirty seven per cent of hostel residents with a neurotic disorder had visited hospital in the past 12 months as an out-patient for a physical complaint; 13% had done so for a mental problem. *(Table 5.18)*

Service use profile

Looking at the whole range of services, from the GP (primary care) to hospital in-patient stays or out-patient visits (secondary care), it can be seen that over half (56%) of hostel residents had some form of secondary care in the past 12 months, while a third just had contact with a GP; only 11% had not used any service. Analysis of the characteristics of those

not receiving any services showed that this group tended to have neither physical or mental long-standing illnesses, nor to be alcohol or drug dependent, suggesting that they probably had no need of medical services. *(Table 5.19)*

Informants with a neurotic disorder were asked some questions to look at service provision under the Care Programme Approach. A third (35%) of hostel residents with a neurotic disorder said they had a key worker, 12% did not know whether they had or not; 54% did not have a key worker. A social worker was the key-worker for almost half of those with a key-worker (44%); among the remainder, no-one reported having a Community Psychiatric Nurse (CPN), Occupational Therapist (OT), Psychologist, Psychiatrist or GP as their key worker - all opted for the 'other' category. The key-worker was seen at least once a month for 90% of people, and for most (54%), contact was much more frequent - at least once a week. Nine per cent of hostel residents with a neurotic disorder knew they had a care manager, 14% did not know and the remainder said they did not have a care manager (data not shown).

Treatment

Information on medication generally taken for mental conditions, and the receipt of counselling or therapy, was collected for all hostel residents. Thirty two per cent of those with a neurotic disorder and 11% of those without such a disorder were taking some form of CNS drug while 14% and 1% respectively were having counselling or therapy. Overall, 40% of those with a disorder were receiving some treatment. Anti-depressant drugs were being taken by 12% of those with a neurotic disorder and 1% of those with no neurotic disorder. Eight per cent of hostel residents with a neurotic disorder were taking hypnotics and anxiolytics, as were 3% of those found to have no neurotic disorder. Among adults identified as having a neurotic disorder in the private household survey only 12% were having any form of treatment (9% any medication, 6% any counselling or therapy). *(Table 5.20)*

5.7 Economic activity and finances

Economic activity

Economic activity among hostel residents follows an entirely different pattern to that found among the private household population; only 12% of men and 18% of women resident in hostels were employed compared with 75% and 63% respectively in private households. Among the non-working hostel population, roughly equal proportions of men were unemployed and economically inactive, while a far higher proportion of the women were economically inactive. A quarter of men reported being permanently unable to work compared with 7% of women; women were far more likely to be 'looking after the home or family'. Major variations in economic activity were not found by neurotic disorder; the main difference was that more of those with a disorder were intending to look for work but temporarily sick, compared with those without a disorder. *(Table 5.21)*

Hostel residents with a neurotic disorder who were not working, but were not retired, were asked why they were not working; 20% said the way they were feeling made work impossible, 18% said that a physical health problem made work impossible and 19% said that their current housing circumstances made it impossible to keep a paid job; 18% said they had not found a suitable job. Of the 33 people who said the way they were feeling made work impossible, 58% thought that all work would be impossible while 25% could do sheltered work and 17% could do part-time work (data not shown). Forty five per cent of hostel residents who were not working, not retired, and who felt they could do some work were currently looking for work; 23% were not looking, but had looked since their last job, and 31% had not looked since their last job. *(Table 5.22)*

Finances

Given the relatively low level of economic activity among hostel residents, it is not surprising that receipt of state benefits was considerably higher among this group than among the private household population. Three quarters of all hostel residents were in receipt of some state benefit; almost two thirds (64%) were receiving Income Support. Variations in receipt of benefits according to neurotic disorder were found only with respect to Sickness Benefit which was being claimed by 10% of those with a neurotic disorder compared with 2% of those with no disorder. *(Table 5.23)*

In addition to collecting information about receipt of state benefits, informants were asked about other sources of income. While 63% of those in hostels relied entirely on state benefits, 13% had benefits and some alternative source of income. Twelve per cent received income but no benefits and a further 12% of respondents received neither state benefits nor income from another source. The majority of those without benefit or income were permanently unable to work (64%); almost half (48%) were aged 45 or over. However 18% fell into the youngest age group, 16-24 years, and it is possible that these were the very youngest hostel dwellers who were too young to register as state benefit claimants (tables not shown). *(Table 5.24)*

The median weekly income among all hostel dwellers was £40-£59; four out of five respondents received less than £100 per week taking account of finances from all sources. *(Table 5.25)*

5.8 Social functioning

Social networks

Some difference was apparent between hostel residents with and without a neurotic disorder with regard to primary support group size; that is the number of adults informants felt close to. A primary support group of 3 people or fewer is indicative of social isolation and is a risk factor for psychiatric morbidity. Over a quarter (27%) of hostel residents with a neurotic disorder had a primary support group of three or fewer people, compared with 19% of those with no neurotic disorder. Among both groups of hostel residents, the proportions with the smallest size primary support group were far higher than among the private household population; among hostel dwellers with no neurotic disorder, only 7% had a primary support group of 3 or fewer adults, compared with 13% among those with a neurotic disorder. *(Table 5.26)*

More detailed information was collected about who people felt close to - this covered family members respondents did and did not live with, and other people resident or not resident at the same address. Although people live in close proximity to others in a hostel environment, three quarters of hostel residents were not living with any other family member and only 14% were living with another adult family member. Half of those with a neurotic disorder and 37% of those with no disorder felt close to no-one who lived at their address. Outside of the hostel, respondents were more likely to have friends or relatives that they felt close to. However, about a quarter of hostel residents said they had no close relatives outside the hostel and a quarter had no close friends. *(Table 5.27)*

Social activities

Hostel residents were asked whether they attended four types of club in their leisure time. Few people attended these places; 6% went to day centres, but only 1% attended each of clubs for people with physical or mental health problems; 13% attended another type of social club. *(Table 5.28)*

5.9   Stressful life events

Respondents were questioned about their experience of each of 11 stressful life events during the past 6 months; these questions were taken from the private household survey. In addition, due to the particular circumstances of homeless people, a question was added about moving home. Sixty one per cent of those with a neurotic disorder and 35% of those with no disorder had moved home and had to find new accommodation in the past 6 months. This life event is excluded from analysis which presents the number of stressful life events respondents had experienced, for comparability with the private household population.

In the private household population, 38% of adults with a neurotic disorder and 17% of those without a disorder had experienced two or more of the 11 stressful life events; among hostel residents the corresponding proportions were 65% and 32%. The experience of stressful life events is one of the areas where greatest differences were observed between hostel residents with and without neurotic disorders. Looking at individual stressful life events, big differences were found with regard to the break-up of a marriage or relationship. This had affected 41% of those with a neurotic disorder compared with 12% of those with no disorder. Over a quarter (28%) of hostel residents with a neurotic disorder had experienced problems with the police involving a court appearance, as had 12% of those with no neurotic disorder; only 2% of people interviewed in the private household survey had this experience. *(Tables 5.29 & 5.30)*

Table 5.1 Distribution of psychotic disorders by classification criteria

Hostel residents

Criteria for inclusion	Percentage	Cumulative percentage
Assessed by SCAN		
Definite: SCAN positive	4	4
Assessed by case study		
Almost certain:	2	6
Fairly certain:	1	8
Little certainty:	1	8
Not psychotic	3	11
Not assessed		
Screen positive on PSQ only; assumed to be non psychotic	21	32
No need to assess		
No psychotic disorder	68	100
Base	*530*	*530*

* Case studies looked at self reported long standing psychotic illness; the duration of episode; doctor's diagnosis of psychotic complaint as reported by informant; use of antipsychotic medication or injections & dosage; outcome of PSQ ; use of mental health services; the use of alcohol and drugs, and alcohol dependence

Table 5.2   Prevalence of psychiatric morbidity by three classification criteria

Hostel residents

Type of disorder	No hierarchy applied	After applying hierarchical rules 1*	After applying hierarchical rules 2**
Any psychotic disorder^	**8%**	**8%**	**8%**
Mixed anxiety and depressive disorder	14%	14%	14%
Depressive episode	12%	11%	11%
Generalised Anxiety Disorder	12%	9%	4%
Phobic disorders	10%	9%	4%
Obsessive- Compulsive Disorder	6%	5%	2%
Panic disorder	4%	3%	3%
Any neurotic disorder^^	**41%**	**38%**	**38%**
Bases	*530/ 499*	*530/ 499*	*530/ 499*

*   Psychosis trumps any neurotic disorder

**   Hierarchy as applied in Private Household Survey i.e. psychosis, severe depressive episode, moderate depressive
      episode, panic disorder, OCD, mild depressive episode, social phobia, agoraphobia, GAD, specific isolated phobia, mixed anxiety and depressive
      disorder

^   Base for psychoses = 530, ie all residents

^^   Base for neuroses = 499, ie excludes residents whose information was obtained by proxy

Table 5.3   Prevalence of alcohol dependence*

Hostel residents

Number of affirmative responses to the 12 alcohol dependence questions**	Percentage	Cumulative percentage
12	2	2
11	2	3
10	1	4
9	2	6
8	3	8
7	1	10
6	1	11
5	1	12
4	1	14
3	2	16
2	4	20
1	4	24
0	76	100
Base	*499*	*499*

*   A score of 3 or more = alcohol dependence

     A score of 7 or more = severe alcohol dependence

**   see appendix B

Table 5.4   Prevalence of drug dependence*

Hostel residents

Category of drug	Percentage
Dependence on ...	
Cannabis	8
Hypnotics	3
Stimulants	3
Hallucinogens inc Ecstasy	1
Other drugs	3
Dependent on cannabis only	5
Dependent on cannabis & other drugs	3
Dependent on non-cannabinoids	3
Dependent on any drug	**11**
Base	*499*

*   Adults were defined as dependent on a drug if they had taken it
     every day for two weeks or more in the past year, and they had
     taken the drug more than prescribed, without prescription or to get
     high. Informants could be dependent on more than one drug

Table 5.5   Socio—demographic characteristics by type of disorder

Hostel residents

	Psychosis	Neurotic disorders	Neither psychotic nor neurotic disorders	Severe Alcohol dependence (7+)	Drug dependence	All
	%	%	%	%	%	%
Sex						
Men	81	68	70	88	90	70
Women	19	32	30	12	10	30
Age						
16-24	14	36	35	28	59	33
25-34	24	28	28	19	28	28
35-44	25	16	10	12	10	14
45-54	16	12	13	24	2	12
55-64	21	8	15	17	-	13
Ethnicity						
White	74	78	75	80	82	76
West Indian/ African	13	15	16	9	13	15
Asian/ Oriental	-	1	1	2	-	1
Other	13	6	8	9	4	7
Marital status						
Married		8	8	0	-	7
Cohabiting	2	5	6	5	7	5
Single	73	60	67	67	82	65
Widowed	-	3	0	-	-	2
Divorced	20	16	12	24	7	15
Separated	5	7	6	4	5	6
Family unit type						
Couple, no children	2	5	5	5	4	5
Couple & child(ren)	-	8	9	0	3	8
Lone parent & child(ren)	3	9	10	-	-	9
One person only	95	77	75	95	93	78
Adult with parents	-	0	0	-	-	0
Adult with one parent	-	-	0	-	-	0
Qualifications						
A level or higher	26	18	19	17	8	18
GCSE/ O level	11	27	21	7	23	22
Other	2	8	12	5	7	10
None	61	47	47	71	61	49
Employment status						
Working full-time	-	10	12	2	4	10
Working part-time	-	3	2	1	3	3
Unemployed	26	39	37	46	61	37
Economically inactive	74	48	49	52	32	50
Base	*41*	*190*	*281*	*48*	*48*	*530*

Table 5.6 Alcohol drinking status by neurotic disorder

Hostel residents

	Neurotic disorder		No neurotic disorder		All	
	%		%		%	
Current drinker*	75		76		76	
Ex - drinker	15	25	12	23	14	24
Always non - drinker	10		11		10	
Base	189		281		470	

* Includes those who drink only very occasionally

Table 5.7 Alcohol consumption level by neurotic disorder and sex

Hostel residents

Alcohol consumption level	Men					Women					All				
	Neurotic disorder		No neurotic disorder		All	Neurotic disorder		No neurotic disorder		All	Neurotic disorder		No neurotic disorder		All
	%		%		%	%		%		%	%		%		%
Abstainer*	20	28	22	32	21	37	48	28	50	31	25	34	24	38	24
Occasional drinker	8		10		9	11		22		18	9		14		12
Light	34		30		32	22		28		26	30		29		30
Moderate	9		15		12	7		14		11	8		14		12
Fairly heavy	5		7		6	9		5		6	6		6		6
Heavy	3	30	2	23	3	2	25	1	8	1	3	27	2	19	2
Very heavy	21		14		17	12		3		7	18		10		14
Base	127		189		316	60		84		144	189		281		470

Note: additional "All" aggregate figures: Men All 30/26, 30; Women All 49/14; All 36/22.

* Includes informants who had not had an alcoholic drink in the past twelve months

69

Table 5.8   Symptoms of alcohol dependence by neurotic disorder

Hostel residents

Symptoms reported	Neurotic disorder	No neurotic disorder	All
	Percentage experiencing symptom		
Woke up next day unable to remember what done while drinking	24	14	18
Skipped meals	25	12	18
Kept on drinking after promised myself not to	20	9	14
Woke sweating due to drinking	13	9	11
Once started drinking, difficult to stop before became completely drunk	17	6	11
Hands shook a lot	12	7	9
Deliberately tried to cut down/ stop but unable	14	6	9
Needed drink so badly, thought of nothing else	12	7	9
Had strong drink in morning to get over effect of previous night's drinking	14	5	8
Stayed drunk for several days	9	7	8
Need more alcohol than used to for same effect	13	4	7
Often had alcoholic drink first thing in morning	8	5	6
Any of above	**31**	**20**	**24**
Alcohol dependence*	22	11	16
Severe alcohol dependence**	13	7	9
Base	*189*	*281*	*470*

*   3 or more symptoms

**   7 or more symptoms

Table 5.9   Symptoms of alcohol dependence: symptomatic behaviour, loss of control and binge drinking by neurotic disorder

Hostel residents

Symptom and score	Neurotic disorder	No neurotic disorder	All
	%	%	%
Binge drinking			
0	91	93	92
1	9	7	8
Symptomatic behaviour			
0	70	81	76
1	6	7	7
2	7	2	4
3	2	3	2
4	5	3	4
5	1	1	1
6	3	-	1
7	6	3	4
(2–7 total)	24	12	17
Loss of control			
0	76	88	83
1	6	4	5
2	6	1	3
3	4	7	6
4	8	0	3
(2–4 total)	18	8	12
Base	*189*	*281*	*470*

70

Table 5.10   Use of drugs by age and sex

Hostel residents

Drug(s) taken	Age			All
	16 -24	25 - 34	35 - 64	
Men	*Percentage using each drug**			
Cannabis	56	29	4	25
Stimulants	25	7	3	10
Amphetamines	22	5	3	8
Cocaine/ crack	10	6	1	4
Hallucinogens inc. Ecstasy	19	4	0	6
Hallucinogens/ psychedelics	13	3	0	4
Ecstasy	11	3	0	4
Opiates	8	6	3	5
Heroin	6	4	3	4
Other opiates including methadone	5	4	3	4
Solvents	5	1	0	1
Any drug	57	31	6	26
Base	*80*	*102*	*142*	*324*
Women	*Percentage using each drug**			
Cannabis	26	14	[1]	19
Stimulants	8	0	[-]	4
Amphetamines	8	0	[-]	4
Cocaine/ crack	3	0	[-]	2
Hallucinogens inc. Ecstasy	13	0	[-]	8
Hallucinogens/ psychedelics	9	0	[-]	5
Ecstasy	6	0	[-]	4
Opiates	4	0	[-]	2
Heroin	4	0	[-]	2
Other opiates including methadone	2	0	[-]	1
Solvents	2	0	[-]	1
Any drug	33	14	[1]	23
Base	*85*	*32*	*[29]*	*146*

Table 5.11   Use of drugs by neurotic disorder

Hostel residents

Drug(s) taken	Neurotic disorder	No neurotic disorder	All
	*Percentage using each drug**		
Cannabis	34	16	23
Stimulants	16	3	8
Amphetamines	13	3	7
Cocaine/crack	7	1	4
Hallucinogens			
inc. Ecstasy	12	3	6
Hallucinogens/			
psychedelics	8	2	4
Ecstasy	6	2	4
Hypnotics	9	4	6
Sleeping tablets	7	2	4
Tranquilisers	7	4	5
Opiates	8	2	4
Heroin	7	1	4
Other opiates			
including methadone	6	1	3
Solvents	2	1	1
Any drug	36	18	25
Base	*189*	*281*	*470*

* Users had taken the drug more than prescribed, without prescription or to get high. They had used the drug in the past year, and more than 5 times in their lifetime. Informants may have taken more than one type of drug.

Table 5.13   Cigarette smoking by neurotic disorder

Hostel residents

Cigarette smoking	Neurotic disorder		No neurotic disorder		All	
	%		%		%	
Non-smoker	16		21		19	
Ex-smoker	13		14		14	
Light smoker	10		12		11	
Moderate smoker	22	71	22	65	22	68
Heavy smoker	38		31		34	
Base	*189*		*281*		*470*	

Table 5.12   Drug dependence (as measured by regularity of use) by neurotic disorder

Hostel residents

Drug(s) dependent on	Neurotic disorder	No neurotic disorder	All
	*Percentage with drug dependence**		
Cannabis	12	6	9
Stimulants	5	1	3
Amphetamines	4	1	2
Cocaine/crack	3	0	1
Hallucinogens			
inc. Ecstasy	1	1	1
Hallucinogens/			
psychedelics	1	0	0
Ecstasy	-	0	0
Hypnotics	4	2	3
Sleeping tablets	2	1	2
Tranquilisers	3	2	2
Opiates	5	1	3
Heroin	4	1	2
Other opiates			
including methadone	2	0	1
Solvents	0	-	0
Any drug	17	7	11
Base	*189*	*281*	*470*

* Adults were defined as dependent on a drug if they had taken it every day for two weeks or more in the past year, and they had taken the drug more than prescribed, without prescription or to get high. Informants could be dependent on more than one drug

Table 5.14   Self reported physical and mental long-standing illness by neurotic disorder

Hostel residents

	Neurotic disorder	No neurotic disorder	All
	%	%	%
No long standing illness	38	63	53
Physical illness only	42	31	36
Physical and mental illness	9	4	6
Mental illness only	11	2	6
Base	*189*	*281*	*470*

Table 5.15 Percentage of residents with long-standing physical complaints by sex

Hostel residents

Physical complaint	Men			Women			All adults		
	Neurotic disorder	No neurotic disorder	All	Neurotic disorder	No neurotic disorder	All	Neurotic disorder	No neurotic disorder	All
	Percentage with each complaint								
Musculo–skeletal complaints	**23**	**10**	**16**	**20**	**9**	**14**	**22**	**10**	**15**
Arthritis/rheumatism/fibrositis	8	4	6	8	2	4	8	4	5
Back & neck problems/ slipped disk	6	4	5	6	5	6	6	4	5
Other problems of bones/joints/ muscles	10	3	6	7	2	4	9	2	5
Respiratory system complaints	**12**	**9**	**10**	**12**	**11**	**12**	**12**	**10**	**11**
Bronchitis/emphysema	0	1	1	-	-	-	0	0	0
Asthma	4	8	6	11	10	11	6	9	8
Hayfever	4	-	2	0	0	0	3	0	1
Other respiratory complaints	3	-	1	2	0	1	3	0	1
Heart/ circulation complaints	**9**	**10**	**10**	**8**	**4**	**6**	**9**	**8**	**8**
Stroke and heart complaints	3	5	4	8	4	6	4	5	4
Blood pressure complaints	5	6	5	-	-	-	3	4	4
Blood vessel complaints	3	4	3	6	-	2	4	2	3
Nervous system complaints	**10**	**10**	**10**	**2**	**2**	**2**	**7**	**8**	**8**
Migraine	2	3	2	2	1	2	2	2	2
Other nervous system complaints	5	6	6	-	-	-	4	4	4
Epilepsy	3	2	2	-	1	0	2	2	2
Digestive system complaints	**12**	**3**	**6**	**9**	**3**	**5**	**11**	**3**	**6**
Stomach complaints & ulcers	11	2	5	6	-	2	9	1	4
Large & small intestine complaints	-	1	0	1	0	1	0	1	0
Other digestive complaints	1	-	0	2	2	2	1	1	1
Other complaints									
Eye complaints	9	6	7	3	0	1	7	4	5
Endocrine disorders	7	3	5	-	-	-	5	2	3
Skin complaints	3	3	3	2	4	3	3	3	3
Neoplasms (and benign lumps or cysts)	1	1	1	8	2	3	3	1	2
Genito- urinary system complaints	-	-	-	6	2	4	2	1	1
Ear complaints	2	3	2	-	-	-	1	2	2
Blood disorders	0	-	0	0	-	0	0	-	0
Infectious and parasitic diseases	-	0	0	-	-	-	-	0	0
Any physical complaint	**53**	**40**	**45**	**53**	**40**	**45**	**51**	**35**	**41**
Base	*129*	*195*	*324*	*60*	*86*	*146*	*189*	*281*	*470*

73

Table 5.16 Access to a doctor by presence of neurotic disorder

Hostel residents

Access to a doctor	Neurotic disorder	No neurotic disorder	All
	%	%	%
If feeling unwell is there a doctor or medical centre you could go to?			
yes	91	97	94
no	7	2	4
don't know	2	1	1
Registered with a doctor?			
yes	93	92	92
no	7	6	7
don't know	-	2	1
Base	*189*	*281*	*470*

Table 5.17 GP consultations by presence of neurotic disorder and sex

Hostel residents

Type of consultation	Neurotic disorder	No neurotic disorder	All
	*Percentage consulting GP**		
Men			
Consulted GP in past 2 weeks for any reason	31	19	24
Consulted GP in past 12 months for physical complaint	76	57	63
Consulted GP in past 12 months for mental complaint	50	14	28
Consulted GP in past 12 months for any complaint	87	60	71
Base	*129*	*195*	*324*
Women			
Consulted GP in past 2 weeks for any reason	40	31	34
Consulted GP in past 12 months for physical complaint	78	71	74
Consulted GP in past 12 months for mental complaint	64	23	40
Consulted GP in past 12 months for any complaint	81	75	77
Base	*60*	*86*	*146*
All adults			
Consulted GP in past 2 weeks for any reason	34	23	27
Consulted GP in past 12 months for physical complaint	76	59	66
Consulted GP in past 12 months for mental complaint	55	16	32
Consulted GP in past 12 months for any complaint	85	65	73
Base	*189*	*281*	*470*

* Consultations in the past 12 months refer to those made on the informant's own behalf

Table 5.18   Percentage of people with neurotic disorders who had been in–patients or out–patients in the past year and reason for hospital stay or visit

Hostel residents

Hospital stay or visit for	In-patient stay		Out-patient visit	
	%		%	
Physical problem	19		30	
Mental problem	-	31	6	43
Both physical and mental problem *	5		7	
Don't know	7		-	
No such stay or visit	64		52	
Don't know whether stay or visit	5		5	
Base	*189*		*189*	

*   Includes more than one stay or visit for different problems, or one visit for both types of problem

Table 5.19   Profile of GP use, in–patient stays and out–patient visits during the past year by neurotic disorder

Hostel residents

Services received	Neurotic disorder	
	%	
None	11	
GP only	33	
GP and out - patient visit	23	
GP and in - patient stay	11	
GP and in - patient stay & out - patient visit	18	56
Out patient visit only	1	
Out - patient visit & in - patient stay	1	
In - patient stay only	2	
Base	*189*	

Where data on in-patient stays and out-patient visits were missing, respondents are categorised with regard only to GP use

Table 5.20   Proportion of people taking each type of CNS medication and having counselling or therapy by disorder

Hostel residents

Type of medication or therapy	Neurotic disorder	No neurotic disorder	All
	Percentage having medication or receiving therapy		
Type of medication:			
Analgesics	**15**	**6**	**9**
Antidepressant drugs	**12**	**1**	**5**
Tricyclic antidepressants	6	1	3
Serotonin reuptake inhibitors	6	0	2
Hypnotics and anxiolytics	**8**	**3**	**5**
Hypnotics	6	2	4
Anxiolytics	4	0	2
Drugs used in psychosis and related conditions	**5**	**1**	**3**
Antipsychotic drugs	5	1	3
Antiepileptics	**2**	**2**	**2**
Drugs used in treatment of substance dependence	**2**	**0**	**1**
Any CNS drugs	**32**	**11**	**19**
Any counselling or therapy	**14**	**1**	**6**
Any psychiatric treatment, medication or therapy	**40**	**11**	**23**
Base	*189*	*281*	*470*

Table 5.21   Economic activity in the past 7 days by neurotic disorder and sex

Hostel residents

	Men			Women			All		
	Neurotic disorder	No neurotic disorder	All	Neurotic disorder	No neurotic disorder	All	Neurotic disorder	No neurotic disorder	All
	%	%	%	%	%	%	%	%	%
Employed									
Employed - at work	7	13	11	24	12	17	12	13	13
Employed - away from job	1	1	1	1	2	1	1	1	1
Employed (total)	8	14	12	25	14	18	13	14	14
Unemployed									
Waiting to start job already obtained	-	1	1	2	-	1	1	1	1
Looking for work	40	39	40	11	22	18	31	34	33
Intending to look, temporarily sick	7	2	4	7	2	4	7	2	4
Unemployed (total)	47	42	45	20	24	23	39	37	38
Economically inactive									
Permanently unable to work	22	26	24	11	4	7	19	19	19
Full time education	1	6	4	0	10	6	1	7	5
Keeping house	2	2	2	25	34	30	9	11	10
Retired	0	3	2	-	-	-	0	2	1
Other	19	7	12	18	13	15	19	9	13
Economically inactive (total)	44	44	44	54	61	58	48	48	48
Base	*129*	*195*	*324*	*60*	*85*	*145*	*189*	*281*	*470*

Table 5.22   Whether looking for work if not working

Hostel residents who were not retired who felt they could do some work

Work seeking status	Neurotic disorder
	%
Currently looking	45
Not looking, although has looked since last job	23
Hasn't looked since last job	31
Base	*125*

(Not looking subtotal: 55)

**Table 5.23 Receipt of State Benefits
by neurotic disorder**

Hostel residents

Type of benefit	Neurotic disorder	No neurotic disorder	All
Percentage receiving benefit*			
Income Support	63	64	64
Child Benefit	11	14	13
Invalidity pension, benefit or allowance	11	10	10
One parent Benefit (in addition to child Benefit)	3	6	5
Unemployment Benefit	3	7	5
Sickness Benefit	10	2	5
Disability Living Allowance	2	4	3
Mobility Allowance	0	4	2
Old Age pension	3	0	1
War Disablement pension	2	1	1
Severe Disablement Allowance	0	2	1
Family Credit	1	1	1
Invalid Care Allowance	1	0	1
Other	9	2	5
Any State Benefit	**79**	**74**	**76**
Base	*189*	*281*	*470*

* Figures for specific benefits represent the minimum percentage
   receiving benefit as questions were not answered by 2% - 8% of adults

Table 5.24   Receipt of State Benefits and other sources of income by neurotic disorder and sex

Hostel residents

In receipt of:	Men			Women			All		
	Neurotic disorder	No neurotic disorder	All	Neurotic disorder	No neurotic disorder	All	Neurotic disorder	No neurotic disorder	All
	%	%	%	%	%	%	%	%	%
State Benefits only; no other source of income	68	62	64	52	65	60	63	63	63
State Benefits and other source of income*	13	9	10	23	15	18	16	11	13
No State Benefits; other source of income only	8	15	12	6	18	13	7	16	12
No State Benefits or other sources of income	11	14	13	19	2	9	14	11	12
Base	*129*	*195*	*324*	*60*	*86*	*146*	*189*	*281*	*470*

* Respondents were asked about receipt of earned income/salary, income from self-employment and income from any other source

Table 5.25   Personal gross income by neurotic disorder

Hostel residents

Yearly income	Weekly income	Neurotic disorder		No neurotic disorder		All	
		%		%		%	
No income		**4**		**1**		**2**	
Less than £1000	Less than £20	4		4		4	
£1000 - £1999	£20 - £39	19		18		18	
£2000 - £2999	£40 - £59	30	79	27	78	28	78
£3000 - £3999	£60 - £79	21		21		21	
£4000 - £4999	£80 - £99	5		9		7	
£5000 - £5999	£100 - £119	2		5		4	
£6000 - £6999	£120 - £139	1		3		2	
£7000 - £7999	£140 - £159	1	8	2	13	2	11
£8000 - £8999	£160 - £179	3		2		2	
£9000 - £9999	£180 - £199	1		1		1	
£10000 - £10999	£200 - £219	3		2		3	
£11000 - £11999	£220 - £239	2		0		1	
£12000 - £12999	£240 - £259	0	6	0	3	0	4
£13000 - £13999	£260 - £279	1		-		0	
£14000 - £14999	£280 - £299	-		-		-	
£15000 or more	£300 or more	1		2		1	
Don't know		**2**		**2**		**2**	
Median weekly income		£40 - £59		£40 - £59		£40 - £59	
Base		*189*		*281*		*470*	

Table 5.26   Size of primary support group by neurotic disorder

Hostel residents

Number of adults in primary support group	Neurotic disorder	No neurotic disorder	All
	%	%	%
0 - 3	27	19	22
4 - 8	31	28	29
9 or more	42	53	49
Base	*189*	*281*	*470*

Table 5.27 Extent of social networks by neurotic disorder

Hostel residents

Type and size of social network	Neurotic disorder	No neurotic disorder	All
	%	%	%
Other family at address?			
No - living alone	77	75	76
Yes - child(ren) only, living as lone parent	9	10	10
Yes - living with other adult family member(s), with or without child(ren)	14	14	14
Adults at same address that feel close to			
0	50	37	42
1	18	26	23
2	15	8	11
3	5	6	6
4 or more	11	23	18
Relatives not at same address that feel close to			
0	26 ⎤	21 ⎤	23 ⎤
1	14 ⎟ 60	14 ⎟ 43	14 ⎟ 50
2	19 ⎦	8 ⎦	12 ⎦
3	6	10	9
4	8	7	7
5	5	8	7
6	7	6	7
7 or more	14	25	20
Friends not at same address that feel close to			
0	24 ⎤	26 ⎤	25 ⎤
1	12 ⎟ 45	11 ⎟ 46	12 ⎟ 46
2	9 ⎦	9 ⎦	9 ⎦
3	10	6	8
4	7	10	9
5	7	6	7
6	10	6	8
7 or more	20	25	23
Base	*189*	*281*	*470*

Table 5.28 Places visited in leisure time for social activities by neurotic disorder

Hostel residents

Type of place	Neurotic disorder	No neurotic disorder	All
	Percentage visiting		
Day centre	3	7	6
Club for people with physical health problems	2	0	1
Club for people with mental health problems	1	0	1
Any other types of social club	12	14	13
Base	*189*	*281*	*470*

Table 5.29 The proportion of adults with each stressful life event by neurotic disorder

Hostel residents

Type of stressful life event	Neurotic disorder	No neurotic disorder	All
	percentage with each stressful life event		
Break up of marriage/ relationship	41	12	24
Seeking work unsuccessfully	35	35	35
Valuable possessions lost/ stolen	34	10	19
Serious problem with close friend	30	10	18
Problems with police - court	28	12	19
Serious illness of close relative	19	13	16
Major financial crisis	19	6	11
Serious personal illness	18	12	14
Death of other relative	11	15	13
Death of close relative	10	3	6
Made redundant from job	10	7	8
Any of the above	**89**	**70**	**78**
Moved home	61	35	46
Base	*189*	*281*	*470*

Table 5.30   Number of stressful life events in past 6 months by neurotic disorder

Hostel residents

Number of stressful life events	Neurotic disorder		No neurotic disorder		All	
	%		%		%	
0	11		30		22	
1	23		39		32	
2	18		17		18	
3	19	65	6	32	11	45
4 or more	29		8		17	
Base	*189*		*281*		*470*	

6 Residents of private sector leased accommodation

Summary

Prevalence of psychiatric morbidity

- The four most prevalent neurotic symptoms among PSLA residents were fatigue, sleep problems, irritability and worry; proportions ranged from 49% for fatigue to 37% for worry.

- Thirty five per cent of the sample had a score of 12 or above on the CIS-R including 27% with scores of 18 or more.

- 1 in 7 PSLA residents were found to have mixed anxiety and depressive disorder and 1 in 8 had depressive episode with about half of those with a depressive episode being in the severe category.

- The prevalence of psychosis among the PSLA sample was estimated at 2%.

- Three per cent of residents were defined as alcohol dependent.

- The prevalence of dependence on non-cannabinoid drugs among PSLA residents was 1%.

Use of alcohol, drugs and tobacco

- Almost a quarter (24%) of adults with a neurotic disorder living in PSLA were non-drinkers.

- Drug use was more prevalent among those with a neurotic disorder compared with those without (21% and 13% respectively).

- Sixty three per cent of those with a neurotic disorder were smokers, compared with 40% of those with no neurotic disorder.

Long-standing illness, treatment and service use

- Over half (54%) of those with a neurotic disorder had a long-standing physical illness and 11% self-reported a long-standing mental complaint.

- Antidepressant drugs were being taken by 5% of those with a neurotic disorder and 3% were taking hypnotics or anxiolytics.

- In the past 12 months, 42% and 6% of respondents with and without a neurotic disorder had consulted a GP for a mental complaint.

Economic, financial and social circumstances

- Seventy two per cent of those with a neurotic disorder had no source of income other than state benefits.

- Over a quarter (28%) of those with a neurotic disorder had a primary support group of three or fewer people, compared with just 9% of those with no neurotic disorder.

- Almost a third (32%) of PSLA residents with a neurotic disorder felt close to no other adults at their address.

- Sixty one per cent of those with, and 29% of those without a neurotic disorder had experienced 2 or more stressful life events in the 6 months prior to interview.

6.1 Introduction

The first part of this chapter shows the prevalence of psychosis, neurotic disorders, alcohol and drug dependence among homeless people, mostly families, temporarily housed in private sector leased accommodation. Of all the four samples of homeless people described in this report, it is this sample which is likely to be most similar to people identified in the private household survey who were living in rented accommodation, especially those renting from Local Authorities or Housing Associations. The second part of the chapter gives a description of the PSLA sample in terms of:

- use of alcohol, drugs and tobacco
- self-reports of long-standing physical and mental health problems
- contact with health services and treatment for mental health problems
- economic activity
- social functioning
- experience of recent stressful life events

The main focus of the analysis of these topics is the investigation of how they are associated with psychiatric morbidity.

6.2 Prevalence of psychiatric morbidity

Neurotic symptoms and disorders

The method of assessing neurotic symptomatology among those living in private sector leased accommodation was identical to that for hostel residents, ie, the interpretation of responses to the revised Clinical Interview Schedule (CIS-R)[2]. Eighty five percent (239 out of 268) were able and willing to complete this interview schedule.

The four most prevalent neurotic symptoms were fatigue, sleep problems, irritability and worry (excluding worry about physical health). The proportions of respondents experiencing these symptoms in the week before interview ranged from 49% for fatigue to 37% for worry. The next most frequently occurring symptoms were depression and depressive ideas, each affecting about a quarter of residents. Even the least prevalent neurotic symptoms - panic and worry about physical health - were found among 12% of informants.

The list of 14 neurotic symptoms in descending order of prevalence, shown in Figure 6.1, is very similar to that found in the private household survey, although each neurotic symptom was more prevalent among this group of homeless people. *(Figure 6.1)*

The distribution of the sum of the scores from all sections of the CIS-R, presented in Figure 6.2, shows that just over a third of the sample, 35%, had a score of 12 or above; scores which represent a neurotic heath problem. This proportion was two and a half times that found in the sample of the private household survey, 14%. The proportion of PSLA residents with scores of 18 or over, 27%, was nearly identical to that found among hostel residents, 28%. *(Figure 6.2)*

When diagnostic algorithms were applied to the CIS-R data, 1 in 7 PSLA residents were found to have mixed anxiety and depressive disorder and 1 in 8 had depressive episode with about half of those with a depressive episode being in the severe category. However, unlike hostel residents, the most prevalent of the phobic disorders among those living in private sector leased accommodation was specific isolated phobia comprising 4% of the 7% who had phobic disorders. *(Figure 6.3)*.

Although residents who fulfilled several diagnostic criteria are represented in each group, comorbid neurotic disorders were not common, affecting 11% of the sample overall including 9% with 2 neurotic disorders. *(Figure 6.4)*

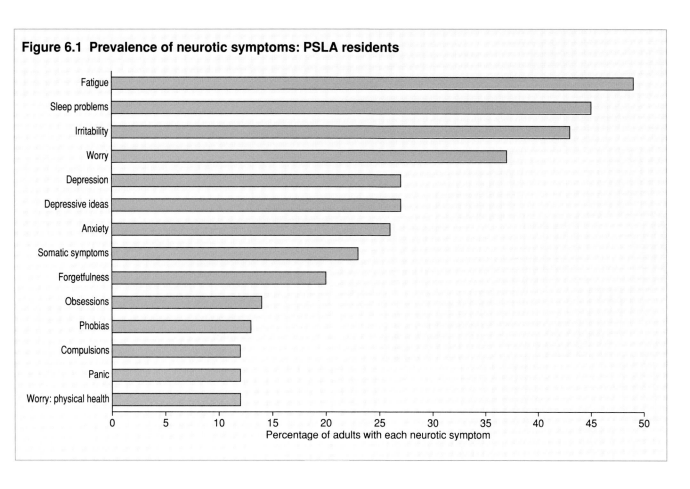

Figure 6.1 Prevalence of neurotic symptoms: PSLA residents

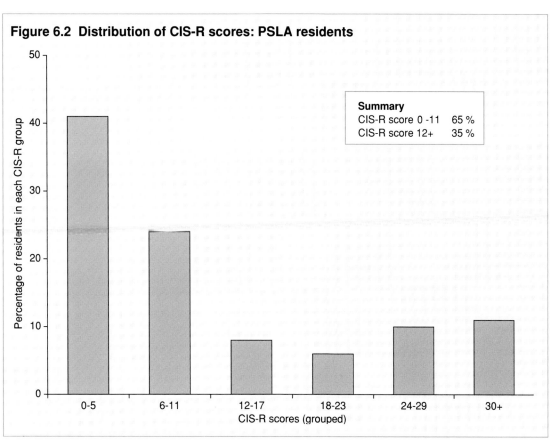

Figure 6.2 Distribution of CIS-R scores: PSLA residents

Summary
CIS-R score 0 -11   65 %
CIS-R score 12+   35 %

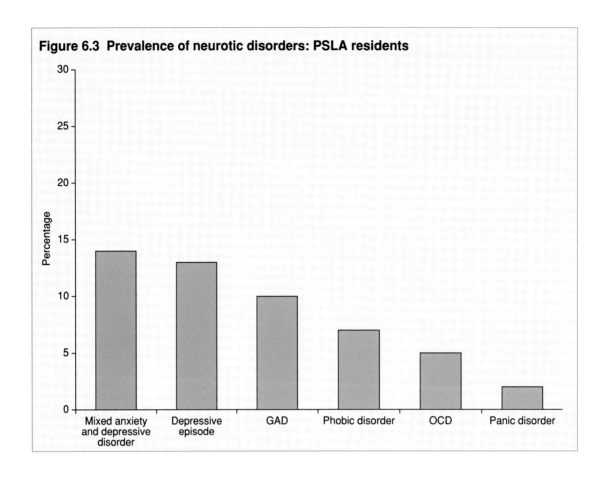

Figure 6.3 Prevalence of neurotic disorders: PSLA residents

As expected the distributions of CIS-R and GHQ12 score were similar, with 42% of the sample having a score of 4 or more including 10% with a maximum score of 12. *(Figure 6.5)*

Psychotic disorders

Chapter 2 of this report gives a detailed account of how psychosis was assessed for all four samples of homeless people. A fifth of the sample satisfied at least one of the sift criteria for psychosis: self-reports of psychosis, the use of antipsychotic medication, or an affirmative response to one of the sections of the Psychosis Screening Questionnaire. After consideration of the results of SCAN interviews, and the evaluation by expert psychiatric epidemiologists of descriptive vignettes, the prevalence of psychosis among the PSLA sample was estimated at 2%. *(Table 6.1)*

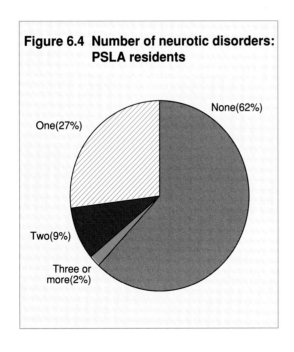

Figure 6.4 Number of neurotic disorders: PSLA residents

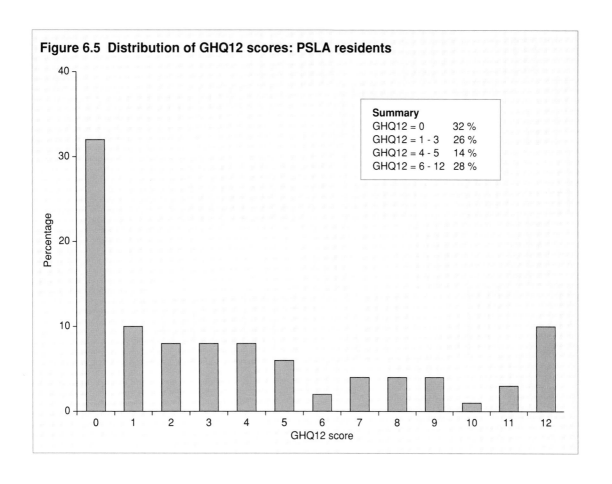

Figure 6.5 Distribution of GHQ12 scores: PSLA residents

Summary
GHQ12 = 0   32 %
GHQ12 = 1 - 3   26 %
GHQ12 = 4 - 5   14 %
GHQ12 = 6 - 12   28 %

Co-occurrence of psychiatric disorders

The prevalence rates of psychosis and each neurotic disorder have so far been presented without the application of any hierarchical rules. In summary, 2% of PSLA residents had psychosis and 38% had a neurotic disorder. When psychosis is treated as trumping any neurotic disorder, the overall prevalence of neurotic disorders hardly changes, falling by 2% to 36%. However, when a hierarchy is imposed within the group of neurotic disorders the prevalence of depressive episode hardly changes but the proportion of residents with Generalised Anxiety Disorder (GAD), phobia or Obsessive Compulsive Disorder (OCD) decrease by at least a half reflecting the lower position of these disorders in the hierarchy. *(Table 6.2)*

Alcohol and drug dependence

Three per cent of PSLA residents were defined as alcohol dependent, a rate more similar to that found in private households (5%) than among hostel residents (16%). *(Table 6.3)*

The prevalence of drug dependence among PSLA residents was 1% for non-cannabinoid drugs, rising to 7% when dependence on cannabis was included. (As the assessment of drug dependence was based on regularity of use, and no other factors, the level of cannabis dependence may be overstated.) *(Table 6.4)*

6.3 Socio-demographic characteristics by type of disorder

Because of the small numbers of those in the sample with psychosis, alcohol and drug dependence, differences in the socio-demographic characteristics of PSLA residents are examined by whether they were assessed as having a neurotic disorder or no psychiatric disorder, that is neither neurosis nor psychosis. Table 6.5 shows that the two groups were not that dissimilar. The neurotic group seemed to have a slighter higher proportion of women, young adults and lone parents. *(Table 6.5)*

The following sections (6.4-6.9) present data on the use of alcohol, drugs and tobacco, self-reported long-standing illnesses, use of services, social networks and stressful life events for adults living in private sector leased accommodation with and without a neurotic disorder . Those with a psychotic disorder are excluded from analysis throughout these sections.

6.4 Use of alcohol, drugs and tobacco

Use of alcohol

This section reports on current drinking status and reasons for stopping drinking alcohol. It then looks at the amount of alcohol people were consuming and at symptoms of alcohol dependence.

Almost a quarter (24%) of adults with a neurotic disorder living in PSLA were categorised as non-drinkers at the time of interview, as were almost a third (31%) of those having no neurotic disorder. Among both groups, most of the non-drinkers had always been non-drinkers. Only 9% of those living in PSLA were consuming levels of alcohol above the recommended sensible level, with no difference between those with and without a neurotic disorder. This proportion is less than half that found among the hostel population, and among adults in private households, although it should be remembered that women tend to have lower levels of alcohol

consumption than men, and that 63% of the PSLA sample was female. Given the comparatively low levels of alcohol consumption, it is not surprising that alcohol dependence was not found to be a major problem among those in PSLA; 4% of respondents were found to be alcohol dependent using the private household survey definition and 2% fulfilled the more stringent criteria for severe alcohol dependence. *(Tables 6.6, 6.7, 6.8 and 6.9)*

Use of drugs

Drug use was more widespread among adults living in PSLA than in the general population, and was more prevalent among those with a neurotic disorder compared with those without (21% and 13% respectively reported using any drug). Dependence on non-cannabinoid drugs was recorded for 3% of PSLA residents with a neurotic disorder, but for none of those with no neurotic disorder. *(Tables 6.10 and 6.11)*

Use of tobacco

Cigarette smoking was associated with having a neurotic disorder among residents of PSLA, as in the private household population, and in contrast to the hostel sample. Sixty three per cent of those with a neurotic disorder were smokers compared with 40% of those with no neurotic disorder; 28% and 12% respectively were described as heavy smokers. *(Table 6.12)*

6.5 Self-reported illness

Major differences were found between PSLA residents with and without a neurotic disorder in the reporting of long-standing illnesses. While 24% of those with no neurotic disorder had a long-standing illness, the corresponding proportion among those with a neurotic disorder was 60%. Over half (54%) of those with a neurotic disorder had a long-standing physical illness and 11% self-reported a long-standing mental complaint. Twenty three per cent of adults with no neurotic disorder had a long-standing physical complaint; none reported a mental complaint. *(Table 6.13)*

About a third of PSLA residents with a long-standing physical illness had a respiratory system complaint; such complaints affected 11% of all PSLA residents compared with 7% of adults in private households. There were some differences between those with and without a neurotic disorder in the prevalence of specific complaints, for example, 13% of those with a neurotic disorder had asthma, compared with 4% of those with no such disorder. The level of blood disorders was notably high, affecting 7% of PSLA residents with a neurotic disorder, compared with 1% of those with no neurotic disorder and 1% of all adults in the private household survey. *(Table 6.14)*

6.6   Use of services and treatment

GPs

Over 95% of PSLA residents with and without a neurotic disorder knew of a doctor or medical centre they could go to if necessary, and were registered with a doctor.

Forty two per cent of PSLA residents with a neurotic disorder and 16% of those with no such disorder consulted a GP in the previous 2 weeks for any reason. In the past 12 months, 42% and 6% of respondents with and without a neurotic disorder had consulted a GP for a mental complaint. Although consultations for mental disorders were notably higher than among the private household population, they were lower than among hostel residents, even though women, who consult the GP more than men, were dominant in the PSLA sample while the hostel population was predominantly male. *(Tables 6.15 and 6.16)*

Hospitals

None of the PSLA residents with a neurotic disorder had in the past 12 months been an in-patient for a mental problem; 3% had visited a hospital as an out-patient for a mental problem. In relation to physical health problems, 12% had been an inpatient and 45% attended hospital as an out-patient.

The service use profile of PSLA residents with a neurotic disorder was very similar to that among hostel residents; in the past year 55% had experienced some form of secondary care, one third had used only a GP and 12% had used no service. *(Tables 6.17 and 6.18)*

Informants with a neurotic disorder were asked some questions to look at service provision under the Care Programme Approach; only 6% reported having a key-worker and no respondents were aware of having a care manager (data not shown).

Treatment

Information on medication generally taken for mental conditions was collected for all PSLA residents. Eighteen per cent of those with a neurotic disorder and 5% of those without such a disorder were taking some form of CNS drug and 2% of those with a neurotic disorder were having counselling or therapy. Antidepressant drugs, mainly tricyclic antidepressants, were being taken by 5% of those with a neurotic disorder, and hypnotics or anxiolytics by 3%. This level of treatment is similar to that found for adults in the private household survey and is lower than among hostel residents. Notably, a smaller proportion of PSLA residents with a neurotic disorder were receiving counselling or therapy compared with those in the private household survey (1% compared with 6%). *(Table 6.19)*

6.7   Economic activity and finances

Economic activity

Economic activity among PSLA residents varied more by sex than by neurotic disorder and overall figures disguise the very different positions for women and men. Forty per cent of all residents were looking after the house and family (61% of women and 5% of men); the second largest group were looking for work (51% of men and 11% of women). Among women in PSLA a higher proportion of those with a neurotic disorder were looking for work (16%) compared with those without a neurotic disorder (7%).

The reasons for not working among PSLA residents who were not working and not retired, differed from those among other groups of homeless people - 19% did not want a paid job, a category that did not feature among other groups. One in ten said the way they were feeling made work impossible compared with 20% of those in hostels. *(Tables 6.20 and 6.21)*

Finances

The majority of PSLA residents (77%) were in receipt of some state benefits; a slightly higher proportion among those with a neurotic disorder (84%) compared with adults with no such disorder (73%). The two most commonly received benefits were Child Benefit, received by 51%, and Income Support (48%). *(Table 6.22)*

Seventy two per cent of those with a neurotic disorder had no source of income other than state benefits as did 61% of those with no disorder; 11% of PSLA residents reported receiving no state benefits or other sources of income. Those in the latter group included all respondents in full-time education, while about half of the group were looking for work. *(Table 6.23)*

The median weekly income among all PSLA residents was £60-£79; 73% of those with a neurotic disorder and 66% of those with no neurotic disorder received less than £100 per week taking account of finances from all sources. Although median weekly income was higher than among hostel residents, it should be remembered that many respondents in PSLA

had to provide for children. *(Table 6.24)*

6.8 Social functioning

Social networks

Major differences were apparent between PSLA residents with and without a neurotic disorder with regard to primary support group size; that is the number of adults informants felt close to. Over a quarter (28%) of those with a neurotic disorder had a primary support group of three or fewer people, compared with just 9% of those with no neurotic disorder. In contrast, among the hostel population, those with no disorder were not so dissimilar from their counterparts with a neurotic disorder in terms of the proportion with a small primary support group, 27% and 19% respectively. *(Table 6.25)*

A quarter of adults living in PSLA identified as having a neurotic disorder were lone parents compared with 15% of those with no neurotic disorder. Only 12% of residents of PSLA were living alone at their address and this did not vary according to neurotic disorder. This compares with 76% of hostel residents. Almost a third (32%) of PSLA residents with a neurotic disorder felt close to no other adults at their address, compared with 18% of those with no disorder. Among adults living with other adult family members, 37% of those with, and 29% of those without a neurotic disorder felt close to no-one in their family (data not shown). *(Table 6.26)*

Social activities

Respondents were asked whether they attended four types of club in their leisure time; 2% went to day centres, 2% attended clubs for people with physical health problems, no-one went to a club for people with mental health problems and 9% attended another type of social club. *(Table 6.27)*

6.9 Stressful life events

Respondents were questioned about their experience of each of 11 stressful life events during the past 6 months; these questions were taken from the private household survey. In addition, a question was added about moving home. Forty eight per cent of those in PSLA had moved home and had to find new accommodation in the past 6 months, with little difference between those with and without a neurotic disorder. This life event is excluded from analysis which presents the number of stressful life events respondents had experienced, for comparability with the private household population.

Among PSLA residents the number of stressful life events experienced varied considerably according to neurotic disorder; 61% of those

with, and 29% of those without a neurotic disorder had experienced 2 or more stressful life events in the 6 months prior to interview. These findings were closer to those for hostel residents than adults living in private households.

Some stressful life events were notably more prevalent among those with neurotic disorders. For example, problems with the police which involved a court appearance had been experienced by 14% of those with a neurotic disorder, compared with 2% of those with no neurotic disorder. A quarter of those with a neurotic disorder had experienced a serious personal illness in the last 6 months as had 9% of PSLA residents who did not have a neurotic disorder. *(Tables 6.28 and 6.29)*

Table 6.1 Distribution of psychotic disorders by classification criteria

PSLA residents

Criteria for inclusion	Percentage	Cumulative percentage
Assessed by SCAN		
Definite: SCAN positive	1	1
Assessed by case study		
Almost certain:	1	2
Fairly certain:	-	2
Little certainty:	0	2
Not psychotic	1	3
Not assessed		
Screen positive on PSQ		
only; assumed to be non-psychotic	17	20
No need to assess		
No psychotic disorder	80	100
Base	*268*	*268*

* Case studies looked at self reported long standing psychotic illness; the duration of episode; doctor's diagnosis of psychotic complaint as reported by informant; use of anti psychotic medication or injections & dosage; outcome of PSQ; use of mental health services; the use of alcohol and drugs, and alcohol dependence

Table 6.2   Prevalence of psychiatric morbidity by three classification criteria

PSLA residents

Type of disorder	No hierarchy applied	After applying hierarchical rules 1*	After applying hierarchical rules 2**
Any psychotic disorder	**2%**	**2%**	**2%**
Mixed anxiety and depressive disorder	14%	14%	14%
Depressive episode	13%	13%	13%
Generalised Anxiety Disorder	10%	10%	4%
Phobic disorders	7%	6%	3%
Obsessive- Compulsive Disorder	5%	5%	2%
Panic disorder	2%	2%	2%
Any neurotic disorder^^	**38%**	**36%**	**36%**
*Bases^*	*268/239*	*268/239*	*268/239*

*   Psychosis trumps any neurotic disorder

**   Hierarchy as applied in Private Household Survey i.e. psychosis, severe depressive episode, moderate depressive episode, panic disorder, OCD, mild depressive episode, social phobia, agoraphobia, GAD, specific isolated phobia, mixed anxiety and depressive disorder

^   Base for psychoses = 268, ie all residents

^^   Base for neuroses = 239, ie excludes residents whose information was obtained by proxy

Table 6.3   Prevalence of alcohol dependence *

PSLA residents

Number of affirmative responses to the 12 alcohol dependence questions**	Percentage	Cumulative percentage
12	1	1
11	-	1
10	0	1
9	-	2
8	1	2
7	-	2
6	-	2
5	1	2
4	1	3
3	1	3
2	1	4
1	2	7
0	93	100
Base	*239*	*239*

*   A score of 3 or more = alcohol dependence
     A score of 7 or more = severe alcohol dependence

**   See appendix B

Table 6.4   Prevalence of drug dependence*

PSLA residents

Category of drug	Percentage
Dependence on ...	
Cannabis	6
Hypnotics	1
Stimulants	0
Hallucinogens inc Ecstasy	-
Other drugs	1
Dependent on cannabis only	6
Dependent on cannabis & other drugs	1
Dependent on non-cannabinoids	1
Dependent on any drug	**7**
Base	*239*

*   Adults were defined as dependent on a drug if they had taken it every day for two weeks or more in the past year, and they had taken the drug more than prescribed, without prescription or to get high. Informants could be dependent on more than one drug.

Table 6.5 Socio–demographic characteristics by type of disorder

PSLA residents

	Neurotic disorder	No neurotic disorder	All*
	%	%	%
Sex			
Men	28	45	37
Women	72	55	63
Age			
16-24	39	37	36
25-34	42	31	36
35-44	15	20	18
45-54	3	9	7
55-64	1	3	2
Ethnicity			
White	69	58	57
West Indian/ African	18	25	22
Asian/ Oriental	8	6	10
Other	3	12	12
Marital status			
Married	37	46	45
Cohabiting	13	9	10
Single	34	34	32
Widowed	2	-	1
Divorced	7	5	5
Separated	7	6	7
Family unit type			
Couple, no children	5	4	6
Couple & child(ren)	45	50	49
Lone parent & child(ren)	25	15	18
One person only	12	12	11
Adult with parents	6	13	10
Adult with one parent	8	5	6
Qualifications			
A level or higher	20	23	20
GCSE/ O level	22	21	20
Other	20	18	17
None	40	38	43
Employment status			
Working full-time	11	12	12
Working part-time	10	9	8
Unemployed	25	30	25
Economically inactive	54	49	55
Base	*88*	*147*	*268*

* Includes proxy informants plus four people with psychosis

Table 6.6 Alcohol drinking status by neurotic disorder

PSLA residents

	Neurotic disorder	No neurotic disorder	All
	%	%	%
Current drinker*	75	69	71
Ex - drinker	8 ⎤ 24	6 ⎤ 31	6 ⎤ 28
Always non - drinker	16 ⎦	26 ⎦	22 ⎦
Base	*88*	*147*	*234*

* Includes those who drink only very occasionally

Table 6.7 Alcohol consumption level by neurotic disorder

PSLA residents

Alcohol consumption level	Neurotic disorder	No neurotic disorder	All
	%	%	%
Abstainer*	24 ⎤ 43	32 ⎤ 48	29 ⎤ 46
Occasional drinker	18 ⎦	16 ⎦	17 ⎦
Light	43	34	37
Moderate	6	8	7
Fairly heavy	5 ⎤	6 ⎤	6 ⎤
Heavy	- ⎥ 8	1 ⎥ 10	0 ⎥ 9
Very heavy	3 ⎦	3 ⎦	3 ⎦
Base	*87*	*144*	*234*

* Includes informants who had not had an alcoholic drink in the past twelve months

Table 6.8 Symptoms of alcohol dependence by neurotic disorder

PSLA residents

Symptoms reported	Neurotic disorder	No neurotic disorder	All
	Percentage experiencing symptom		
Woke up next day unable to remember what done while drinking	2	7	6
Skipped meals	3	4	4
Once started drinking, difficult to stop before became completely drunk	4	4	4
Woke sweating due to drinking	1	2	2
Kept on drinking after promised myself not to	2	3	3
Need more alcohol than used to for same effect	2	2	2
Deliberately tried to cut down/ stop but unable	1	2	2
Needed drink so badly, thought of nothing else	2	2	2
Had strong drink in morning to get over effects of previous night's drinking	2	1	2
Stayed drunk for several days	1	1	1
Hands shook a lot	2	1	1
Often had alcoholic drink first thing in morning	2	0	1
Any of above	**5**	**8**	**7**
Alcohol dependence*	4	3	4
Severe alcohol dependence**	1	2	2
Base	*88*	*147*	*234*

* 3 or more symptoms
** 7 or more symptoms

Table 6.9 Symptoms of alcohol dependence: symptomatic behaviour, loss of control and binge drinking by neurotic disorder

PSLA residents

Symptom and score	Neurotic disorder	No neurotic disorder	All
	%	%	%
Binge drinking			
0	99	99	99
1	1	1	1
Symptomatic behaviour			
0	95	92	93
1	1	5	4
2	1	1	1
3	1	-	0
4	1	2	1
5	- (4)	- (3)	- (3)
6	-	0	0
7	1	0	0
Loss of control			
0	96	96	96
1	1	1	1
2	2	1	1
3	- (3)	0 (3)	0 (3)
4	1	2	1
Base	*88*	*147*	*234*

Table 6.10 Use of drugs by neurotic disorder

PSLA residents

Drug(s) taken	Neurotic disorder	No neurotic disorder	All
*Percentage using each drug**			
Cannabis	18	13	15
Stimulants	6	2	3
Amphetamines	4	2	3
Cocaine/crack	1	-	0
Hallucinogens inc. Ecstasy	1	2	2
Hallucinogens/ psychedelics	-	2	1
Ecstasy	1	1	1
Hypnotics	2	0	1
Sleeping tablets	2	-	1
Tranquilisers	2	0	1
Opiates	2	-	1
Heroin	2	-	1
Other opiates including methadone	2	-	1
Any drug	21	13	16
Base	*88*	*147*	*234*

* Users had taken the drug more than prescribed, without prescription or to get high. They had used the drug in the past year, and more than 5 times in their lifetime. Informants may have taken more than one type of drug

Table 6.11 Drug dependence (as measured by regularity of use) by neurotic disorder

PSLA residents

Drug(s) dependent on	Neurotic disorder	No neurotic disorder	All
*Percentage with drug dependence**			
Cannabis	10	5	6
Stimulants	1	-	0
Amphetamines	1	-	0
Cocaine/crack	-	-	-
Hallucinogens inc. Ecstasy	-	-	-
Hallucinogens/psychedelics	-	-	-
Ecstasy	-	-	-
Hypnotics	1	-	1
Sleeping tablets	1	-	1
Tranquilisers	1	-	1
Opiates	2	-	1
Heroin	2	-	1
Other opiates including methadone	2	-	1
Any non-cannabinoid drug	3	0	1
Any drug	11	5	7
Base	*88*	*147*	*234*

* Adults were defined as dependent on a drug if they had taken it every day for two weeks or more in the past year, and they had taken the drug more than prescribed, without prescription or to get high. Informants could be dependent on more than one drug

93

Table 6.12   Cigarette smoking by neurotic disorder

PSLA residents

Cigarette smoking	Neurotic disorder		No neurotic disorder		All	
	%		%		%	
Non - smoker	22		39		33	
Ex - smoker	15		20		18	
Light smoker	17		9		12	
Moderate smoker	18	63	19	40	19	49
Heavy smoker	28		12		18	
Base	88		147		234	

Table 6.13   Self reported physical and mental long-standing illness by neurotic disorder

PSLA residents

	Neurotic disorder		No neurotic disorder		All	
	%		%		%	
Physical illness only	49		23		33	
Physical and mental illness	5	60	-	24	2	38
Mental illness only	6		1		3	
No long standing illness	40		76		62	
Base	88		147		234	

Table 6.14   Percentage of residents with long-standing physical complaints

PSLA residents

Physical complaint	Neurotic disorder	No neurotic disorder	All
	Percentage with each complaint		
Respiratory system complaints	18	7	11
Bronchitis/emphysema	1	-	0
Asthma	13	4	8
Hayfever	6	2	3
Other respiratory complaints	1	2	2
Musculo- skeletal complaints	13	5	8
Arthritis/rheumatism/fibrositis	1	4	3
Back & neck problems/ slipped disk	6	1	3
Other problems of bones/joints/muscles	7	1	3
Heart/ circulation complaints	9	5	6
Stroke and heart complaints	6	3	4
Blood pressure complaints	8	1	4
Blood vessel complaints	0	0	0
Digestive system complaints	9	3	5
Stomach complaints & ulcers	7	3	4
Large & small intestine complaints	2	-	1
Other digestive complaints	1	-	0
Nervous system complaints	9	2	4
Migraine	5	-	2
Other nervous system complaints	1	1	1
Epilepsy	2	1	1
Other complaints			
Genito- urinary system complaints	3	4	4
Blood disorders	7	1	3
Eye complaints	6	2	3
Endocrine disorders	1	1	1
Skin complaints	1	1	1
Neoplasms (and benign lumps or cysts)	1	1	1
Infectious and parasitic diseases	1	0	1
Ear complaints	-	1	1
Any physical complaint	54	23	35
Base	88	147	234

Table 6.15   Access to a doctor by presence of neurotic disorder

PSLA residents

Access to a doctor	Neurotic disorder	No neurotic disorder	All
	%	%	%
If feeling unwell is there a doctor or medical centre you could go to?			
yes	95	95	95
no	3	4	4
don't know	2	0	1
Registered with a doctor?			
yes	96	94	95
no	4	5	5
Base	*88*	*147*	*234*

Table 6.17   Percentage of people with neurotic disorders who had been in-patients or out-patients in the past year and reason for hospital stay or visit

PSLA residents

Hospital stay or visit for	In-patient stay		Out-patient visit	
	%		%	
Physical problem	12	⎤	43	⎤
Mental problem	-		1	
Both physical &		16		45
mental problem *	0		2	
Don't know	4	⎦	-	⎦
No such stay or visit	76		47	
Don't know whether stay or visit	8		8	
Base	*88*		*88*	

*   Includes more than one stay or visit for different problems, or one stay or visit for both types of problem

Table 6.16   GP consultations by presence of neurotic disorder

PSLA residents

Type of consultation	Neurotic disorder	No neurotic disorder	All
	Percentage consulting GP*		
Consulted GP in past 2 weeks for any reason	42	16	26
Consulted GP in past 12 months for physical complaint	74	61	66
Consulted GP in past 12 months for mental complaint	42	6	20
Consulted GP in past 12 months for any complaint	81	63	70
Base	*88*	*147*	*234*

*   Consultations in the past 12 months refer to those made on the informant's own behalf

Table 6.18   Profile of GP use, in-patient stays and out-patient visits during the past year by neurotic disorder

PSLA residents

Services received	Neurotic disorder
	%
None	12
GP only	33
GP and out-patient visit	32 ⎤
GP and in-patient stay	10
GP and in-patient stay & out-patient visit	6
Out-patient visit only	7 ⎬ 55
Out-patient visit & in-patient stay	1
In-patient stay only	- ⎦
Base	*88*

Where data on in-patient stays and out-patient visits were missing, respondents are categorised with regard only to GP use

Table 6.19 Proportion of people taking each type of CNS medication and having counselling or therapy by disorder

PSLA residents

Type of medication or therapy	Neurotic disorder	No neurotic disorder	All
Percentage having medication or receiving therapy			
Type of medication:			
Analgesics	**10**	**2**	**5**
Antidepressant drugs	**5**	**1**	**2**
Tricyclic antidepressants	4	1	2
Serotonin reuptake inhibitors	1	0	0
Hypnotics and anxiolytics	**3**	**2**	**2**
Hypnotics	1	0	0
Anxiolytics	3	2	2
Drugs used in psychosis and related conditions	**1**	**1**	**1**
Antipsychotic drugs	1	1	1
Antlepileptics	**1**	**0**	**0**
Drugs used in treatment of substance dependence	**0**	**0**	**0**
Any CNS drugs	**18**	**5**	**10**
Any counselling or therapy	**2**	**0**	**1**
Any psychiatric treatment: medication or therapy	**19**	**5**	**11**
Base	*88*	*147*	*234*

Table 6.20 Economic activity in the past 7 days by neurotic disorder and sex

PSLA residents

	Men			Women			All		
	Neurotic disorder	No neurotic disorder	All	Neurotic disorder	No neurotic disorder	All	Neurotic disorder	No neurotic disorder	All
	%	%	%	%	%	%	%	%	%
Employed									
Employed - at work	[6]	20	21	14	12	13	17	16	16
Employed - away from job	[0]	4	4	5	6	6	4	5	5
(total)	[6]	24	25	19	18	19	21	21	21
Unemployed									
Looking for work	[8]	57	51	16	7	11	21	29	26
Intending to look, temporarily sick	[2]	-	2	2	1	1	4	0	2
(total)	[10]	57	53	18	8	12	25	29	28
Economically inactive									
Keeping house	[2]	5	5	60	62	61	45	36	40
Permanently unable to work	[5]	6	10	2	-	1	7	2	4
Full time education	[-]	4	3	-	9	5	-	7	4
Other	[1]	5	4	2	2	2	2	4	3
(total)	[7]	20	22	64	73	69	54	49	51
Base	*24*	*66*	*90*	*63*	*81*	*143*	*88*	*147*	*234*

Table 6.21 Reasons for not working among those with neurotic disorders

PSLA residents who were not working, but were not retired

Why not working?	Neurotic disorder
	%
Way feeling makes work impossible	10
Physical health problem makes work impossible	18
Current housing circumstances make it impossible to keep a paid job	8
Have not found suitable paid job	18
Do not want/ need paid job	19
Other	26
Base	*63*

**Table 6.22   Receipt of State Benefits
by neurotic disorder**

PSLA residents

Type of benefit	Neurotic disorder	No neurotic disorder	All
	*Percentage receiving benefit**		
Child Benefit	56	48	51
Income Support	57	42	48
One parent Benefit (in addition to child Benefit)	11	8	9
Family Credit	4	6	6
Unemployment Benefit	0	5	3
Invalidity pension, benefit or allowance	1	3	2
Old Age pension	0	2	1
Maternity benefit	2	0	1
Other	0	3	2
Any State Benefit	**84**	**73**	**77**
Base	*88*	*147*	*234*

*   Figures for specific benefits represent the minimum percentage
    receiving benefit as questions were not answered by 2% - 8%
    of adults

Table 6.23   Receipt of State Benefits and other sources of income by neurotic disorder and sex

PSLA residents

In receipt of:	Men			Women			All		
	Neurotic disorder	No neurotic disorder	All	Neurotic disorder	No neurotic disorder	All	Neurotic disorder	No neurotic disorder	All
	%	%	%	%	%	%	%	%	%
State Benefits only; no other source of income	[19]	54	61	70	67	68	72	61	65
State Benefits and other source of income*	[1]	4	5	15	17	16	12	12	12
No State Benefits; other source of income only	[4]	23	21	8	5	6	10	13	12
No State Benefits or other sources of income	[-]	19	14	8	10	9	6	14	11
Base	*24*	*66*	*90*	*64*	*81*	*144*	*88*	*147*	*234*

* Respondents were asked about receipt of earned income/salary, income from self-employment and income from any other source

Table 6.24 Personal gross income by neurotic disorder

PSLA residents

Yearly income	Weekly income	Neurotic disorder		No neurotic disorder		All	
		%		%		%	
No income		**5**		**10**		**8**	
Less than £1000	Less than £20	15		10		12	
£1000 - £1999	£20 - £39	21		16		18	
£2000 - £2999	£40 - £59	8	73	15	65	12	68
£3000 - £3999	£60 - £79	22		12		16	
£4000 - £4999	£80 - £99	7		12		10	
£5000 - £5999	£100 - £119	7		9		8	
£6000 - £6999	£120 - £139	6		2		4	
£7000 - £7999	£140 - £159	2	19	2	19	2	19
£8000 - £8999	£160 - £179	2		5		4	
£9000 - £9999	£180 - £199	2		0		1	
£10000 - £10999	£200 - £219	1		1		1	
£11000 - £11999	£220 - £239	-		0		0	
£12000 - £12999	£240 - £259	1	3	-	1	0	2
£13000 - £13999	£260 - £279	-		-		-	
£14000 - £14999	£280 - £299	1		-		0	
£15000 or more	£300 or more	-		2		1	
Don't know		**1**		**4**		**3**	
Median weekly income		£60 -£79		£60 -£79		£60 -£79	
Base		*88*		*147*		*234*	

Table 6.25 Size of primary support group by neurotic disorder

PSLA residents

	Neurotic disorder	No neurotic disorder	All
	%	%	%
0 - 3	28	9	16
4 - 8	42	34	36
9 or more	30	57	48
Base	*88*	*147*	*234*

Table 6.26 Extent of social networks by neurotic disorder

PSLA residents

Type and size of social network	Neurotic disorder	No neurotic disorder	All
	%	%	%
Other family at address?			
No - living alone	12	12	12
Yes - child(ren) only, living as lone parent	25	15	19
Yes - living with other adult family member(s), with or without child(ren)	63	73	69
Adults at same address that feel close to			
0	32	18	23
1	48	46	47
2	13	25	21
3	6	5	5
4 or more	–	7	4
Relatives not at same address that feel close to			
0	12 ⎤	9 ⎤	10 ⎤
1	26 ⎥ 57	6 ⎥ 40	13 ⎥ 46
2	20 ⎦	24 ⎦	22 ⎦
3	15	9	11
4	8	8	8
5	7	8	8
6	2	8	6
7 or more	11	27	21
Friends not at same address that feel close to			
0	20 ⎤	10 ⎤	14 ⎤
1	16 ⎥ 57	11 ⎥ 39	13 ⎥ 46
2	21 ⎦	18 ⎦	19 ⎦
3	6	11	9
4	7	12	10
5	2	4	3
6	9	15	13
7 or more	18	19	18
Base	*88*	*147*	*234*

Table 6.27 Places visited in leisure time for social activities by neurotic disorder

PSLA residents

Type of place	Neurotic disorder	No neurotic disorder	All
	Percentage visiting		
Day centre	3	2	2
Club for people with physical health problems	4	-	2
Club for people with mental health problems	-	-	-
Any other types of social club	5	12	9
Base	*88*	*147*	*234*

Table 6.28 The proportion of adults with each stressful life event by neurotic disorder

PSLA residents

Type of stressful life event	Neurotic disorder	No neurotic disorder	All
	Percentage with each stressful life event		
Seeking work unsuccessfully	35	26	30
Serious problem with close friend	35	6	17
Serious personal illness	26	9	15
Break up of marriage/ relationship	19	13	15
Valuable possessions lost/ stolen	17	10	13
Serious illness of close relative	17	12	14
Major financial crisis	16	5	9
Problems with police- court	14	2	6
Death of other relative	14	15	15
Death of close relative	3	1	2
Made redundant from job	2	7	5
Any of the above	**84**	**64**	**71**
Moved home	51	47	48
Base	*88*	*147*	*234*

Table 6.29 Number of stressful life events in past 6 months by neurotic disorder

PSLA residents

Number of stressful life events	Neurotic disorder	No neurotic disorder	All
	%	%	%
0	16	36	29
1	23	35	30
2	34	19	25
3	9 (61)	8 (29)	9 (41)
4 or more	18	2	8
Base	*88*	*147*	*234*

101

7 Residents of nightshelters

Summary

Prevalence of psychiatric morbidity

- Nearly 60% of homeless people staying in nightshelters had a score at or above (defined as caseness) the threshold value of 4 on the GHQ12; 40% had a score of 6 or more.

- Forty three per cent of nightshelter residents were positive on at least one of the psychosis sift criteria. However, this 43% included 33% who only screened positive because of their answers to the Psychosis Screening Questionnaire.

- Forty four percent of those staying at nightshelters were alcohol dependent. The proportion deemed to have severe alcohol dependence was 31%.

- A quarter of nightshelter residents were dependent on some sort of drug. They tended to be extensive users of non-cannabinoid drugs: heroin or opiates (10%), stimulants (10%), hypnotics (8%) and hallucinogens (5%).

Use of alcohol, drugs and tobacco

- Forty four per cent of those with GHQ12 scores of 4 or more were very heavy drinkers as were 32% of those scoring 0-3 on the GHQ12.

- Forty per cent of nightshelter residents used cannabis and 13% used opiates.

- One in seven residents had injected drugs at some time in their lives.

- All of those with a GHQ12 score of 4 or more were smokers.

Long-standing illness, treatment and service use

- Half the sample reported a longstanding illness with 30%, overall, mentioning a mental complaint.

- The proportion of adults with a GHQ12 score of 4 or more who had seen a GP in the past 12 months for any complaint was 64%. The same proportion reporting having access to a GP.

- One in nine residents had seen a GP, had an in-patient stay and had an out-patient visit in the past 12 months: 15% of cases compared with just 5% of non-cases.

- Almost a quarter (24%) of nightshelter residents with a GHQ12 score of 4 or more were using drugs prescribed for mental condition.

Economic and financial circumstances

- Among those not working, 31% of cases and 12% of non-cases said that the way they were feeling made work impossible.

- Over three quarters of nightshelter residents were receiving state benefits (77%); the majority were in receipt of Income Support - 72% of cases, and 63% of non-cases.

7.1 Introduction

In this chapter the main method of distinguishing between those who had or did not have a mental health problem was the response to the GHQ12. Pilot work showed that it was not viable to ask the CIS-R of people using nightshelters. Thus, it is not possible to present prevalence rates of neurotic disorders for this group. In addition, difficulties in following up those who screened positive for psychosis with a clinical interview means that reliable estimates of psychosis are precluded. Nevertheless, the results of the interview carried out by OPCS interviewers show that 43% of nightshelter residents were positive on at least one of the psychosis sift criteria: self-report of psychosis, prescribed antipsychotic medication or a significant psychotic trait as measured by the Psychosis Screening Questionnaire. However, care needs to be taken in the interpretation of this result as this 43% included 33% who only screened positive because of their answers to the Psychosis Screening Questionnaire. As we have seen in the analysis of hostel and PSLA residents, the majority of these are likely to be false positives.

We were able to collect sufficient data on alcohol and drug dependence to allow analysis on these two topics. Therefore, the characteristics of nightshelter residents are described predominantly in terms of GHQ12 scores and measures of alcohol and drug dependence.[1]

7.2 Prevalence of psychiatric morbidity

GHQ12

Nearly 60% of homeless people staying in nightshelters had a score at or above the threshold value of 4 on the GHQ12 and 40% had a score of 6 or more, (roughly equivalent to scores of 12 or more and 18 or more on the CIS-R)[2]. *(Figure 7.1)*

Alcohol and drug dependence

Alcohol dependence was very prevalent. Forty four percent of those staying in nightshelters had alcohol dependence (defined as a positive response to at least three of the 12 questions describing symptoms and behaviour indicative

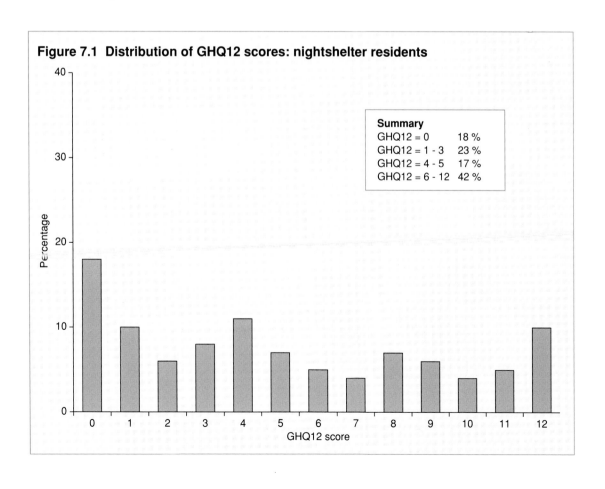

Figure 7.1 Distribution of GHQ12 scores: nightshelter residents

Summary
GHQ12 = 0	18 %
GHQ12 = 1 - 3	23 %
GHQ12 = 4 - 5	17 %
GHQ12 = 6 - 12	42 %

of alcohol dependence). The proportion with 7 or more positive responses, deemed to have severe alcohol dependence was 31%. *(Table 7.1)*

Drug dependence was also fairly widespread among nightshelter residents with 29% dependent on some sort of drug (including cannabis where our measure is likely to be over-inclusive, see Appendix B for details on definitions). Drug dependence among nightshelter residents was different to that among hostel and PSLA residents not only in extent, but also in type. Whereas the latter groups were mainly dependent on cannabis, among those living in nightshelters, comparatively high rates of dependence were found for non-cannabinoid drugs: heroin or opiates (10%), stimulants (10%), hypnotics (8%) and hallucinogens (5%). *(Table 7.2)*

7.3 Socio-demographic characteristics by GHQ12 scores

There were no significant differences in the socio-demographic characteristics of nightshelter residents according to whether they had a score of 0-3 or 4 or more on the GHQ12. *(Table 7.3)*

However, considerable differences were found within the sample when comparing the socio-demographic characteristics of those who had severe alcohol dependence, drug dependence and those with neither problem. Residents who were drug dependent were predominantly young, single, white men who were either unemployed or economically inactive with better educational qualifications than their co-residents. Among those with severe alcohol dependence, 40% were aged 45 or above, 41% were separated or divorced, and 64% had no educational qualifications. *(Table 7.4)*

The following sections (7.4-7.7) present data on use of alcohol, drugs and tobacco, self-reported long-standing illnesses, use of

services, and the economic and financial circumstances of the nightshelter sample; data are shown separately for those who scored 4 or more (cases), and 3 or less (non-cases), on the GHQ12.

7.4 Use of alcohol, drugs and tobacco

Use of alcohol

Only 13% of nightshelter residents were categorised as non-drinkers at the time of interview. The largest proportion of respondents were classified as very heavy drinkers than in any of the other alcohol consumption level categories: 44% of those with GHQ12 scores of 4 or more were very heavy drinkers as were 32% of those scoring 0-3 on the GHQ12. Almost a third (31%) of nightshelter residents were categorised as having severe alcohol dependence, with the proportion slightly higher among cases compared with non-cases. Significant symptoms of alcohol dependence were far more prevalent among the nightshelter population compared with hostel residents. Binge drinking, for example, was recorded for 23% of those in nightshelters compared with 8% of hostel residents and symptomatic behaviour for 46% compared with 17%. The differences in the level of alcohol dependence between cases and non-cases among nightshelter residents were less marked than those between hostel residents with and without a neurotic disorder. *(Tables 7.5, 7.6, 7.7 and 7.8)*

Use of drugs

Drug use among those resident in nightshelters far exceeded the levels found even among hostel residents, a group that was previously shown to use drugs far more extensively than the private household population. Forty per cent of nightshelter residents used cannabis and 13% used opiates; the corresponding proportions among hostel residents were 23% and 4% respectively. Differences in the use of most types of drugs were identified among nightshelter residents in the two GHQ12 groups. However, it is interesting to note that dependence levels were the same for the two groups with regard to many of the drugs. The exceptions were amphetamines and Ecstasy where a higher proportion of non-cases were classified as dependent, and heroin and solvents where a higher proportion of cases had dependence. *(Tables 7.9 and 7.10)*

One in seven nightshelter residents had ever injected drugs:19% of those with a score of 4 or more on the GHQ12 and 8% of non-cases. Within the last month, 12% and 4% respectively had injected drugs (data not shown).

Use of tobacco

Half (53%) of those with a score of 4 or more on the GHQ12 were classified as very heavy smokers, compared with almost a third (31%) of the non-cases. *(Table 7.11)*

7.5 Self-reported illness

Although half the sample reported a long-standing illness, major differences were found between nightshelter residents defined as cases and non-cases. Sixty two per cent of cases had some long-standing illness compared with 26% of non-cases. More specifically, a mental illness was reported by 30% of cases and 8% of non-cases. The overall level of self-reported, long-standing illness among cases in nightshelters was identical to that for hostel residents with a neurotic disorder. Although the latter group reported slightly more physical illness, mental complaints were more prevalent among those in nightshelters (30% in nightshelters compared with 20% in hostels). *(Table 7.12)*

Looking at the types of physical complaints reported, some differences in the prevalence of

musculo-skeletal complaints and respiratory system complaints can be seen between cases and non-cases in nightshelters (18% compared with 10%, and 14% compared with 4% respectively). *(Table 7.13)*

7.6 Use of services and treatment

GPs

Access to a doctor varied notably by GHQ12 score; overall 72% of nightshelter residents knew of a doctor or medical centre they could visit if they were feeling unwell, and 71% said they were registered with a doctor. Among those with a score of 4 or more on the GHQ12, 65% had access to a doctor compared with 81% of those scoring 0-3. For both groups the proportions with access to a doctor were considerably lower than among other groups of homeless adults. *(Table 7.14)*

Despite lower overall access to medical services, the proportion of nightshelter residents having GP consultations in the past two weeks was actually similar to that for hostel residents (29% compared with 27%). Looking at GP consultations over the past 12 months among nightshelter residents is hampered by the fact that the necessary information is missing for one in five residents. Among cases, almost half (48%) had seen a GP about a mental complaint in the past 12 months and for a quarter (24%), we do not know; among the non-cases 14% had made such a consultation and information is unavailable for 11%. The proportion of cases who had seen a GP in the past 12 months for any complaint (64%), is identical to the proportion reporting access to a GP. Additional analysis showed that some of those who reported not presently having access to a GP, had in the past 12 months seen a GP (data not shown). It may be that some nightshelter residents did not visit a GP due to access problems rather than lack of need, however it is not possible to determine this from these data. *(Table 7.15)*

Those who had spoken to a doctor in the past 2 weeks were asked where they had spoken to the

GP; 84% had been to the GP's surgery, or to a health centre, 16% had seen the doctor at a day centre or hostel clinic and 5% had seen a GP somewhere else. *(Table 7.16)*

Hospitals

Information about hospital in-patient stays and out-patient visits was collected for all nightshelter residents. Fifteen per cent of cases had been treated as an in-patient for a mental problem over the past 12 months, as had 8% of non-cases; 15% and 5% respectively had been treated as out-patients for a mental complaint. In-patient stays and out-patient visits for physical health problems were more common than those for mental conditions; 20% of nightshelter residents had been treated as an in-patient, and 34% as an out-patient, for a physical complaint.

Looking at the service use profile of nightshelter residents, it can be seen that secondary care had been received by a higher proportion of cases (61%), than non-cases (49%). One in nine residents had seen a GP, had an in-patient stay and had an out-patient visit in the past 12 months: 15% of cases compared with just 5% of those scoring 0-3 on the GHQ12. *(Tables 7.17 and 7.18)*

Eighteen per cent of nightshelter residents reported having a key worker and 5% did not know whether they had one. There was little difference between the cases and the non-cases. Six per cent had a care manager and 8% did not know (data not shown).

Treatment

Almost a quarter (24%) of nightshelter residents with a GHQ12 score of 4 or more were using drugs prescribed for mental conditions, compared with almost a third (32%) of hostel residents with a neurotic disorder. In both nightshelters and hostels, 11% of those with no evidence of neurotic psychopathology were taking CNS drugs.

Hypnotics and anxiolytics were the most commonly used drugs among cases and non-cases in nightshelters; 13% and 9% respectively were taking this medication. Analgesics were being taken by 11% of cases, compared with just 1% of non-cases. Twelve per cent of cases and 5% of non-cases in nightshelters were having some form of counselling or therapy. *(Table 7.19)*

7.7 Economic activity and finances

Economic activity

The proportion of nightshelter residents who were employed (7%) was half that of hostel residents (14%). A higher proportion of those in nightshelters were unemployed; 61% of cases and 50% of non-cases. Eighteen per cent of nightshelter residents said they were permanently unable to work, with little difference between cases and non-cases; this corresponds almost exactly to the proportion of hostel residents who were permanently unable to work. *(Table 7.20)*

Respondents who were not working, but not retired, were asked why they were not working; 31% of cases and 12% of non-cases said that the way they were feeling made work impossible. Thirty seven per cent said that their current housing circumstances made it impossible to keep a paid job; this finding did not differ between the cases and the non-cases. *(Table 7.21)*

Finances

Over three quarters of nightshelter residents were receiving state benefits (77%); the majority were in receipt of Income Support - 72% of cases, and 63% of non-cases. Nine per cent of respondents were receiving Sickness Benefit and 9% were receiving an Invalidity Pension, benefit or allowance. *(Table 7.22)*

Eighteen per cent of those in nightshelters were receiving neither state benefits, nor had other sources of income. The median weekly income was £40-59 a week among both cases and non-cases. *(Tables 7.23 and 7.24)*

Residents of nightshelters were not asked about their social functioning, or about stressful life events experienced over the last 6 months because the context of the questions was inappropriate.

Notes and references

1. The prevalence and socio-demographic sections are based on all respondents; subsequent sections comparing cases and non-cases exclude the few known cases of psychosis.

2. See Appendix C for details of the comparability study of the two instruments: CIS-R and GHQ12.

Table 7.1   Prevalence of alcohol dependence*

Nightshelter residents

Number of affirmative responses to the 12 alcohol dependence questions**	Percentage	Cumulative percentage
12	9	9
11	3	12
10	1	13
9	2	16
8	6	22
7	9	31
6	2	33
5	4	37
4	4	43
3	1	44
2	3	47
1	8	54
0	46	100
Base	*181*	*181*

* A score of 3 or more = alcohol dependence
   A score of 7 or more = severe alcohol dependence

** See appendix B

Table 7.2   Prevalence of drug dependence*

Nightshelter residents

Category of drug	Percentage
Dependence on ...*	
Cannabis	18
Stimulants	10
Hypnotics	8
Hallucinogens inc Ecstasy	5
Heroin or opiates	10
Solvents	3
Dependent on cannabis only	6
Dependent on cannabis & other drug	11
Dependent on non-cannabinoids	11
Dependent on any drug	**29**
Base	*185*

* Adults were defined as dependent on a drug if they had taken it every day for two weeks or more in the past year, and they had taken the drug more than prescribed, without prescription or to get high. Informants could be dependent on more than one drug

Table 7.3   Socio-demographic characteristics by GHQ12 score

Nightshelter residents

	GHQ12 score		All*
	4 or more	0-3	
	%	%	%
Sex			
Women	10	12	11
Men	90	88	89
Age			
16-24	30	29	29
25-34	31	31	31
35-44	12	11	12
45-54	19	16	18
55-64	7	14	10
Ethnicity			
White	97	83	91
West Indian/ African	2	11	5
Asian/ Oriental	-	-	-
Other	1	6	3
Marital status			
Married	2	-	1
Cohabiting	1	1	1
Single	69	77	73
Widowed	1	1	1
Divorced/ separated	27	21	24
Qualifications			
A level or higher	16	23	19
GCSE/ O level	22	24	23
Other	9	9	9
None	53	44	49
Employment status			
Working full-time	2	5	3
Working part-time	4	3	3
Unemployed	58	52	54
Economically inactive	36	41	39
Base	*107*	*74*	*185*

*   Includes four residents with insufficient data on GHQ12

Table 7.4   Socio-demographic characteristics of adults classified as alcohol and drug dependent

Nightshelter residents

	Alcohol dependent (severe)	Drug dependent	Neither alcohol nor drug dependent	All residents
	%	%	%	%
Sex				
Men	96	90	85	89
Women	4	10	15	11
Age				
16-24	35	43	24	29
25-34	20	45	31	31
35-44	5	8	16	12
45-54	28	3	17	18
55-64	12	1	12	10
Ethnicity				
White	100	98	85	91
West Indian/ African	-	1	9	5
Asian/ Oriental	-	-	1	-
Other	-	1	6	3
Marital status				
Married	1	2	1	1
Cohabiting	-	3	-	1
Single	57	83	79	73
Widowed	1	-	1	1
Divorced/ separated	41	12	19	24
Qualifications				
A level or higher	8	13	26	19
GCSE/ O level	19	45	11	23
Other	10	2	10	9
None	64	40	53	49
Employment status				
Working full-time	2	1	5	3
Working part-time	-	-	7	3
Unemployed	53	45	59	54
Economically inactive	45	53	29	39
Base	*57*	*53*	*96*	*185*

Table 7.5 Alcohol drinking status by GHQ12 score

Nightshelter residents

	GHQ12 score		All
	4 or more	0-3	
	%	%	%
Current drinker*	85	87	86
Ex-drinker	9 ⎤	3 ⎤	6 ⎤
Always non-drinker	5 ⎦ 16	9 ⎦ 13	7 ⎦ 13
Base	*99*	*77*	*176*

* Includes those who drink only very occasionally

Table 7.6 Alcohol consumption level by GHQ12 score

Nightshelter residents

Alcohol consumption level	GHQ12 score		All
	4 or more	0-3	
	%	%	%
Abstainer*	15 ⎤ 22	12 ⎤ 20	14 ⎤ 21
Occasional drinker	7 ⎦	8 ⎦	7 ⎦
Light	17	25	21
Moderate	6	8	7
Fairly heavy	8 ⎤	10 ⎤	9 ⎤
Heavy	3 ⎟ 55	5 ⎟ 48	4 ⎟ 52
Very heavy	44 ⎦	32 ⎦	39 ⎦
Base	*99*	*77*	*176*

* Includes informants who had not had an alcoholic drink in the past twelve months

Table 7.7 Symptoms of alcohol dependence by GHQ12 score

Nightshelter residents

Symptoms reported	GHQ12 score		All
	4 or more	0-3	
	Percentage experiencing symptom		
Woke up next day unable to remember what done while drinking	47	45	46
Skipped meals	47	34	42
Kept on drinking after promised myself not to	36	31	33
Once started drinking, difficult to stop before became completely drunk	36	27	32
Had strong drink in morning to get over effects of previous night's drinking	35	30	33
Woke sweating due to drinking	32	22	28
Needed drink so badly, thought of nothing else	28	14	22
Hands shook a lot	26	23	25
Need more alcohol than used to for same effect	26	27	26
Often had alcoholic drink first thing in morning	25	30	27
Stayed drunk for several days	24	21	23
Deliberately tried to cut down/ stop but unable	20	16	19
Any of above	**52**	**55**	**54**
Alcohol dependence*	47	38	43
Severe alcohol dependence**	34	26	31
Base	*99*	*77*	*176*

* 3 or more symptoms

** 7 or more symptoms

Table 7.8   Symptoms of alcohol dependence: symptomatic behaviour, loss of control and binge drinking by GHQ12 score

Nightshelter residents

Symptom and score	GHQ12 score		All
	4 or more	0 - 3	
	%	%	%
Binge drinking			
0	76	79	77
1	24	21	23
Symptomatic behaviour			
0	48	47	48
1	3	11	6
2	6 ⌐	9 ⌐	7 ⌐
3	8	4	6
4	6	4	5
5	9 | 49	9 | 42	9 | 46
6	5	8	7
7	14 ⌐	9 ⌐	12 ⌐
Loss of control			
0	53	63	57
1	8	10	8
2	20 ⌐	11 ⌐	16 ⌐
3	5 | 39	9 | 28	7 | 34
4	14 ⌐	7 ⌐	11 ⌐
Base	*99*	*77*	*176*

Table 7.9   Use of drugs by GHQ12 score

Nightshelter residents

Drug(s) taken	GHQ12 score		All
	4 or more	0-3	
	*Percentage using each drug**		
Cannabis	**44**	**34**	**40**
Stimulants	**24**	**14**	**20**
Amphetamines	19	14	17
Cocaine/crack	12	4	9
Hallucinogens inc. Ecstasy	**18**	**18**	**18**
Hallucinogens/ psychedelics	16	8	13
Ecstasy	11	11	11
Hypnotics	**16**	**13**	**20**
Sleeping tablets	21	11	17
Tranquilisers	19	12	16
Opiates	**16**	**10**	**13**
Heroin	15	7	12
Other opiates including methadone	13	8	11
Solvents	**18**	**11**	**15**
Any drug	**52**	**37**	**46**
Base	*99*	*77*	*176*

*   Users had taken the drug more than prescribed, without prescription or to get high. They had used the drug in the past year, and more than 5 times in their lifetime. Informants may have taken more than one type of drug

Table 7.10 Drug dependence (as measured by regularity of use) by GHQ12 score

Nightshelter residents

Drug(s) dependent on	GHQ12 score		All
	4 or more	0-3	
	*Percentage with drug dependence**		
Cannabis	19	18	18
Stimulants	10	10	10
Amphetamines	3	10	6
Cocaine/crack	8	0	4
Hallucinogens inc. Ecstasy	2	9	5
Hallucinogens/ psychedelics	2	2	2
Ecstasy	1	8	4
Hypnotics	8	7	8
Sleeping tablets	7	3	5
Tranquilisers	5	5	5
Opiates	14	7	11
Heroin	13	7	10
Other opiates including methadone	4	0	2
Solvents	6	1	4
Any non-cannabinoid drug	23	22	23
Any drug	33	24	29
Base	*99*	*77*	*176*

* Adults were defined as dependent on a drug if they had taken it every day for two weeks or more in the past year, and they had taken the drug more than prescribed, without prescription or to get high. Informants could be dependent on more than one drug.

Table 7.11 Cigarette smoking by GHQ12 score

Nightshelter residents

Cigarette smoking	GHQ12 score		All
	4 or more	0-3	
	%	%	%
Non - smoker	0	13	6
Ex - smoker	10	9	10
Light smoker	12	15	14
Moderate smoker	24 (89)	32 (78)	28 (85)
Heavy smoker	53	31	43
Base	*99*	*77*	*175*

Table 7.12 Self reported physical and mental long-standing illness by GHQ12 score

Nightshelter residents

	GHQ12 score		All
	4 or more	0 - 3	
	%	%	%
Physical illness only	32	18	26
Physical and mental illness	14 (62)	2 (26)	9 (47)
Mental illness only	16	6	12
No long standing illness	38	74	53
Base	*99*	*77*	*176*

Table 7.13 Physical long-standing complaints by GHQ12 score

Nightshelter residents

Physical complaint	GHQ12 score		All
	4 or more	0-3	
	Percentage with each complaint		
Musculo-skeletal complaints	**18**	**10**	**14**
Arthritis/rheumatism/ fibrositis	3	4	3
Back & neck problems/ slipped disk	4	2	3
Other problems of bones/ joints/muscles	11	4	8
Respiratory system complaints	**14**	**4**	**10**
Bronchitis/emphysema	2	2	2
Asthma	6	1	4
Hayfever	-	1	0
Other respiratory complaints	6	-	3
Heart/ circulation complaints	**9**	**2**	**6**
Stroke and heart complaints	8	2	6
Blood pressure complaints	-	-	-
Blood vessel complaints	-	-	-
Nervous system complaints	**6**	**4**	**5**
Epilepsy	4	1	3
Migraine	1	1	1
Other nervous system complaints	2	2	2
Digestive system complaints	**3**	**2**	**2**
Stomach complaints & ulcers	3	1	2
Large & small intestine complaints	-	0	2
Other digestive complaints	-	1	0
Other complaints			
Endocrine disorders	5	2	4
Skin complaints	6	-	3
Neoplasms (and benign lumps or cysts)	3	1	2
Infectious and parasitic diseases	3	-	2
Eye complaints	2	1	1
Blood disorders	1	-	0
Ear complaints	0	-	0
Genito- urinary system complaints	-	-	-
Any physical complaint	**46**	**20**	**35**
Base	*99*	*77*	*176*

Table 7.14 Access to a doctor by GHQ12 score

Nightshelter residents

Access to a doctor	GHQ12 score		All
	4 or more	0-3	
	%	%	%
If feeling unwell is there **a doctor or medical centre you could go to?**			
yes	65	81	72
no	32	19	26
don't know	4	-	2
Registered with a doctor?			
yes	64	80	71
no	34	19	27
don't know	2	2	2
Base	*99*	*77*	*176*

Table 7.15 GP consultations by GHQ12 score

Nightshelter residents

Type of consultation		GHQ12 score		All
		4 or more	0-3	
		Percentage consulting GP*		
Consulted GP in past 2 weeks for physical complaint only		17	18	18
Consulted GP in past 2 weeks for mental complaint only		8	5	7
Consulted GP in past 2 weeks for physical and mental complaint together		9	1	6
Consulted GP in past 2 weeks for any reason		33	24	29
		%	%	%
Whether consulted GP in past 12 months for physical complaint	Yes	53	60	56
	No	23	28	25
	Unknown	24	11	19
Whether consulted GP in past 12 months for mental complaint	Yes	48	14	33
	No	28	75	48
	Unknown	24	11	19
Whether consulted GP in past 12 months for any complaint	Yes	64	61	63
	No	12	28	18
	Unknown	24	11	19
Base		*99*	*77*	*176*

* Consultations refer to those made on the informant's own behalf and informants may have had more than one consultation.

Table 7.16   Location of GP consultation

Adults visiting nightshelters who spoke to a doctor on their own behalf in the past 2 weeks

Doctor contacted at:

	Percentage speaking with doctor at each location*
GP surgery/ health centre	84%
Day centre/ hostel clinic	16%
Spoke to GP on telephone	-
Other	5%
Base	*50*

* Percentages total more than 100% as people may have contacted a doctor on more than one occasion, at different locations

Table 7.17   Percentage of people who had been in-patients or out-patients in the past year and reason for hospital stay or visit by GHQ12 score

Nightshelter residents

Reason for stay/visit	In - patient stay			Out - patient visit		
	GHQ12 score			GHQ12 score		
	4 or more	0-3	All	4 or more	0-3	All
	%	%	%	%	%	%
Physical problems	18	11	15	32	30	31
Mental problems	5 ⎤ 34	8 ⎤ 19	7 ⎤ 27	12 ⎤ 47	1 ⎤ 34	7 ⎤ 41
Both physical & mental problems*	10 ⎦	- ⎦	6 ⎦	3 ⎦	4 ⎦	3 ⎦
No such stay or visit	65	80	72	53	66	58
Base	*99*	*77*	*176*	*99*	*77*	*176*

* Includes more than one stay or visit for different problems, or one stay or visit for both types of problem

Table 7.18 Profile of GP use, in-patient stays and out-patient visits during the past year by GHQ12 score

Nightshelter residents

Services received	GHQ12 score		All
	4 or more	0 - 3	
	%	%	%
None	18	27	22
GP only	21	24	22
GP and out - patient visit	17	25	20
GP and in - patient stay	11	7	9
GP and in - patient stay & out - patient visit	15	5	11
Out patient visit only	9	5	7
Out - patient visit & in - patient stay	6	-	4
In - patient stay only	3	7	4
	61	*49*	*56*
Base	*99*	*76*	*175*

Where data on in-patient stays and out-patient visits were missing, respondents are caregorised with regard only to GP use

Table 7.19 Proportion of people taking each type of CNS medication and having counselling or therapy by GHQ12 score

Nightshelter residents

Type of medication or therapy	GHQ12 score		All
	4 or more	0-3	
	Percentage having medication or receiving therapy		
Medication:			
Hypnotics and anxiolytics	**13**	**9**	**11**
Hypnotics	9	6	7
Anxiolytics	5	4	5
Analgesics	**11**	**1**	**6**
Drugs used in treatment of substance dependence	**3**	**4**	**4**
Antiepileptics	**3**	**0**	**2**
Antidepressant drugs	**4**	**4**	**4**
Tricyclic antidepressants	2	4	3
Serotonin reuptake inhibitors	2	0	1
Any CNS drugs	**24**	**11**	**18**
Any counselling or therapy	**12**	**5**	**9**
Any psychiatric treatment, medication or therapy	**31**	**12**	**23**
Base	*99*	*77*	*176*

116

Table 7.20 Economic activity in the past 7 days by GHQ12 score

Nightshelter residents

	GHQ12 score		All
	4 or more	0-3	
	%	%	%
Employed			
Employed - at work	3 ⎤	7 ⎤	5 ⎤
Employed -	⎬ 7	⎬ 7	⎬ 7
away from work	4 ⎦	- ⎦	2 ⎦
Unemployed			
Looking for work	54 ⎤	41 ⎤	48 ⎤
Intending to look,	⎥	⎥	⎥
temporarily sick	6 ⎬ 61	8 ⎬ 50	7 ⎬ 56
Waiting to start job	⎥	⎥	⎥
already obtained	1 ⎦	1 ⎦	1 ⎦
Economically inactive			
Permanently unable			
to work	20 ⎤	16 ⎤	18 ⎤
Full time education	- ⎬ 33	1 ⎬ 43	0 ⎬ 36
Other	13 ⎦	26 ⎦	18 ⎦
Base	*99*	*77*	*176*

Table 7.21 Reasons for not working by GHQ12 score

Nightshelter residents who were not retired who felt they could do some work

Why not working?	GHQ12 score		All
	4 or more	0-3	
	%	%	%
Way feeling makes work impossible	31	12	23
Physical health problem makes work impossible	13	16	14
Current housing circumstances make it impossible to keep a paid job	36	38	37
Have not found suitable paid job	18	30	23
Do not want/ need paid job	2	4	3
Base	*89*	*69*	*158*

Table 7.22 Receipt of State Benefits by GHQ12 score

Nightshelter residents

Type of benefit	GHQ12 score		All
	4 or more	0-3	
	Percentage receiving benefit*		
Income Support	72	63	68
Sickness Benefit	7	12	9
Invalidity pension, benefit or allowance	8	9	9
Disability Living Allowance	1	2	2
Severe Disablement Allowance	3	1	2
Unemployment Benefit	4	4	4
War Disablement pension	2	0	1
Other	1	1	1
Any State Benefit	**79**	**75**	**77**
Base	*99*	*77*	*176*

* Figures for specific benefits represent the minimum percentage receiving benefit as questions were not answered by 2% - 8% of adults

Table 7.23 Receipt of State Benefits and other sources of income by GHQ12 score

Nightshelter residents

In receipt of:	GHQ12 score		All
	4 or more	0-3	
	%	%	%
State Benefits only; no other source of income	71	69	70
State Benefits and other source(s) of income*	7	6	7
No State Benefits; other source(s) of income only	4	7	5
No State Benefits or other source of income	18	17	18
Base	*99*	*77*	*176*

* Respondents were asked about receipt of earned income/salary, income from self-employment and income from any other source

117

Table 7.24 Personal gross income by GHQ12 score

Nightshelter residents

Yearly income	Weekly income	GHQ12 score		All	
		4 or more	0-3		
		%	%	%	
No income		**9**	**12**	**10**	
Less than £1000	Less than £20	5	1	3	
£1000 - £1999	£20 - £39	24	21	23	
£2000 - £2999	£40 - £59	28 ⎱82	27 ⎱76	27 ⎱80	
£3000 - £3999	£60 - £79	18	26	22	
£4000 - £4999	£80 - £99	6	2	4	
£5000 - £5999	£100 - £119	2	-	1	
£6000 - £6999	£120 - £139	-	2	1	
£7000 - £7999	£140 - £159	- ⎱2	3 ⎱5	1 ⎱3	
£8000 - £8999	£160 - £179	1	-	0	
£9000 - £9999	£180 - £199	-	-	-	
£10000 - £10999	£200 - £219	2	1	1	
£11000 - £11999	£220 - £239	-	-	-	
£12000 - £12999	£240 - £259	- ⎱2	0 ⎱4	0 ⎱3	
£13000 - £13999	£260 - £279	-	1	0	
£14000 - £14999	£280 - £299	-	2	1	
£15000 or more	£300 or more	1	-	0	
Don't know		**5**	**2**	**4**	
Median weekly income		£40 - £59	£40 - £59	£40 - £59	
Base		*99*	*77*	*176*	

8 Homeless people sleeping rough using day centres

Summary

Prevalence of psychiatric morbidity

- Fifty seven percent of homeless people who were sleeping rough had a score above the threshold value of 4 on the GHQ12. Overall, nearly a half (47%) had a score of 6 or more. A fifth of the sample had a score of 10, 11 or 12.

- Forty seven per cent of the sample were positive on at least one of the psychosis sift criteria. This proportion is likely to include many false positives as 43% overall only screened positive because of their answers to the Psychosis Screening Questionnaire.

- Half the people interviewed were assessed as alcohol dependent and just over a third, 36%, had severe alcohol dependence.

- Twelve per cent of day centre visitors were dependent on non-cannabinoid drugs.

Use of alcohol, drugs and tobacco

- 47% of cases (those with a GHQ12 score of 4 or more) and 32% of non-cases (GHQ12 score of 0-3) were defined as very heavy drinkers.

- 37% of day centre visitors were found to be drug users.

- Twenty per cent of the sample had injected drugs and 6% had shared injection equipment. Six per cent had injected drugs in the last month.

- Nine in ten homeless adults visiting day centres smoked cigarettes and 46% were heavy smokers.

Long-standing illness, treatment and service use

- Sixty one per cent of people sleeping rough visiting day centres reported a long-standing illness.

- Nineteen per cent of day centre visitors had a respiratory system complaint and 18% had musculo-skeletal complaints. Epilepsy was reported by 6% and stomach complaints by 5%.

- Seventy eight per cent of the sample said they knew of a doctor or medical centre they could visit if they were feeling unwell, yet only 58% were registered with a doctor.

- Two thirds (68%) of day centre visitors reported a GP consultation over the past 12 months, with a wide discrepancy between cases (80%) and non-cases (53%).

- Thirty two per cent of people sleeping rough had been treated as a hospital in-patient during the past 12 months and 38% reported an out-patient visit, predominantly for physical health problems.

- Almost a third of those sleeping rough (31%) had received some form of psychiatric treatment; 47% of cases and 11% of non-cases.

119

Economic and financial circumstances

- A larger proportion of cases than non-cases stated that they were permanently unable to work: 28% compared with 19%.

- Fifty eight per cent of the sample received Income Support; 15% were getting Sickness benefit and 8% had an Invalidity Pension.

8.1 Introduction

The method of differentiating those who had or did not have a mental health problem among homeless people using day centres was identical to that for nightshelter residents: the response to the GHQ12. For this sample, it was even more difficult to follow up those who screened positive for psychosis with a clinical interview . The OPCS interview found that 47% of people sleeping rough using day centres were positive on at least one of the psychosis sift criteria: self report of psychosis, prescribed antipsychotic medication or a significant psychotic trait as measured by the Psychosis Screening Questionnaire. However, this proportion is likely to include many false positives as 43% only screened positive because of their answers to the Psychosis Screening Questionnaire.

Data on alcohol and drug dependence were collected. The prevalence rates of GHQ12 scores, alcohol and drug dependence and the results of the analysis of the key survey topics are presented in the same way in this chapter as for nightshelter residents in the previous chapter.[1]

8.2 Prevalence of psychiatric morbidity

GHQ12

Fifty seven percent of homeless people who were sleeping rough for at least one day in the week prior to interview who were identified in day centres had a score at or above the threshold value of 4 on the GHQ12. Overall, nearly a half (47%) had a score of 6 or more, equivalent to a CIS-R score of 18 or more. At the extreme end of the distribution, a fifth of the sample had a score of 10, 11 or 12. *(Figure 8.1)*

Alcohol and drug dependence

Half the people interviewed were assessed as alcohol dependent and just over a third, 36%, had severe alcohol dependence. *(Table 8.1)*.

Drug dependence was also fairly prevalent among homeless people sleeping rough, with about a quarter dependent on some sort of drug. Our dependence assessment based on regularity of use probably over-estimates cannabis dependence (18%) however it is less likely to over-estimate dependence on non-cannabinoid drugs (12%). Although the level of drug dependence among those in day centres was similar to that for nightshelter residents, those sleeping rough were less likely to be dependent on non-cannabinoid drugs. *(Table 8.2)*

8.3 Socio-demographic characteristics by GHQ12 scores

There were some marked differences in the socio-demographic characteristics of those sleeping rough according to whether they had a score of 0-3 or 4 or above on the GHQ12. Comparing those with scores at or above the threshold score to those below, the higher scorers consisted of proportionately more women (18% compared with 5%) and double the percentage of divorced and separated people (38% compared with 19%). *(Table 8.3)*

Considerable differences were also found within the sample when comparing the socio-demographic characteristics of those who were alcohol dependent, drug dependent and those with neither problem. The profiles of drug and

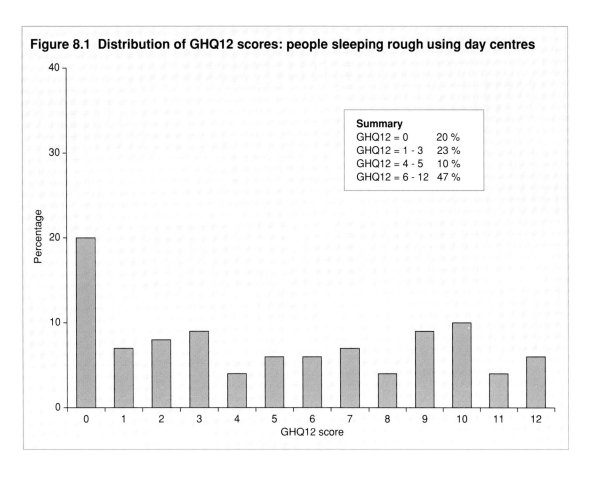

Figure 8.1 Distribution of GHQ12 scores: people sleeping rough using day centres

Summary
GHQ12 = 0   20 %
GHQ12 = 1 - 3   23 %
GHQ12 = 4 - 5   10 %
GHQ12 = 6 - 12 47 %

alcohol dependent adults sleeping rough was similar to that for residents of nightshelters. Those with drug dependence tended to be young, single men whereas among those who were alcohol dependent, 44% were aged 45 or over, 41% were divorced or separated and 73% had no educational qualifications. *(Table 8.4)*

The following sections (8.4-8.7) present data on the use of alcohol, drugs and tobacco, self-reported long-standing illness, the use of services and economic activity for adults included in the day centre sample; data are shown separately for those who scored 4 or more, and 3 or less, on the GHQ12.

8.4 Use of alcohol, drugs and tobacco

Use of alcohol

Only 15% of homeless people sleeping rough were categorised as non-drinkers at the time of interview and the majority of these were ex-

drinkers; only 3% of those interviewed in day centres had always been non-drinkers. Over half (54%) of respondents were found to drink more than the recommended sensible level of alcohol; 47% of cases and 32% of non-cases were defined as very heavy drinkers which corresponds almost exactly to the proportions among nightshelter residents. *(Tables 8.5 and 8.6)*.

Over a third (36%) of adults visiting day centres had severe alcohol dependence. The proportion of adults with severe alcohol dependence among cases was twice that of non-cases,(46% compared with 23%). While the overall level of severe alcohol dependence among this group was very similar to that among nightshelter residents, the contrast between the cases and non-cases was much more marked among those in day centres than among the nightshelter sample. Looking at the components of alcohol dependence, significant symptomatic behaviour was reported for 54% of cases and 43% of non-cases in day centres, loss of control for 51% and 29% respectively and binge drinking for 44% and 32%. Binge drinking and loss of control in particular, were higher among day centre visitors compared with nightshelter residents. *(Tables 8.7 and 8.8)*

Use of drugs

The use of drugs, and dependence on them, was lower among day centre visitors than those resident in nightshelters, although higher than among hostel residents. Overall, 37% of day centre visitors were found to be drug users, with no difference between cases and non-cases. This compares with 46% of nightshelter residents using drugs and notable differences between cases and non-cases among that population.

Misuse of hypnotics and opiates did show some variation between cases and non-cases in the day centre population. Eighteen per cent of cases used opiates and 8% were dependent on these drugs compared with 8% and 4% of non-cases. Dependence on non-cannabinoid drugs affected 14% of day centre cases, and 8% of non-cases. *(Tables 8.9 and 8.10)*

Twenty per cent of day centre visitors had injected drugs and 6% had shared injection equipment. Six per cent had injected drugs in the last month, 1% sharing equipment (data not shown).

Use of tobacco

Nine in ten homeless adults visiting day centres smoked cigarettes and 46% were heavy smokers. There was little variation by GHQ12 score. The pattern differed somewhat from that found for nightshelter residents where a higher proportion of cases, compared with non-cases were heavy smokers (53% and 31% respectively) and where more of the non-cases did not smoke at all (22%). *(Table 8.11)*

8.5   Self-reported illness

Sixty one per cent of people sleeping rough visiting day centres reported a long-standing illness compared with 47% of those resident in nightshelters. There were differences between cases and non-cases although, for physical illnesses, these were not so marked as in the nightshelter population. Thirty per cent of day centre visitors with a GHQ12 score of 4 or more, self-reported a long-standing mental complaint, as did 11% of those with a score of 3 or lower. These figures were very similar to those among nightshelter cases and non-cases. While 54% of day centre visitors had a long-standing physical complaint, the corresponding proportion among nightshelter residents was far lower at 35%. *(Table 8.12)*

Nineteen per cent of day centre visitors had a respiratory system complaint and 18% had musculo-skeletal complaints. Epilepsy was reported by 6% and stomach complaints by 5%. Some differences were found between cases and non-cases, for example 16% and 4% respectively had asthma. However, the differences between this population and the nightshelter population in the prevalence of physical illness are perhaps more noteworthy than those between cases and non-cases in day centres. For example, respiratory complaints affected 10% of those in nightshelters, half the proportion affected in day centres. Digestive system complaints affected 2% of nightshelter residents compared with 9% of day centre visitors. Part of the difference in physical illness between the day centre and nightshelter populations may relate to differences in the age structure of the two groups, the former having fewer people in the youngest age category. *(Table 8.13)*

8.6   Use of services and treatment

GPs

Seventy eight per cent of those interviewed in day centres said they knew of a doctor or medical centre they could visit if they were feeling unwell, however only 58% were registered with a doctor. A similar proportion of cases and non-cases had access to a doctor

(75% and 82% respectively), although a notably higher proportion of cases were registered with a doctor, 66% compared with 48% of non-cases. Compared with the nightshelter population, access rates were similar, but levels of registration were lower for users of day centres. *(Table 8.14)*

The overall rate of GP consultations in the past two weeks for any reason, was identical among people sleeping rough visiting day centres and nightshelter residents, 32%. However differences between cases and non-cases were much more marked in the day centre population; 44% of cases compared with 17% of non-cases had consulted a GP in the two weeks prior to interview.

Two thirds (68%) of day centre visitors reported a GP consultation over the past 12 months, with wide discrepancy between cases (80%) and non-cases (53%). Almost half (47%) of the cases had spoken to the GP about a mental complaint in the past 12 months, as had 14% of non-cases. *(Table 8.15)*

Those who had spoken to a doctor in the past 2 weeks were asked where they had spoken to the GP; 72% had been to the GP's surgery, or to a health centre, 20% had seen the doctor at a day centre or hostel clinic and 4% had spoken to a GP on the telephone. *(Table 8.16)*

Hospitals

Thirty two per cent of day centre visitors had been treated as a hospital in-patient during the past 12 months and 38% reported an out-patient visit over the same period. These findings were similar to those among nightshelter residents. The majority of in-patient stays and out-patient visits were for physical health problems. In-patient stays were reported by a far higher proportion of cases (45%) than non-cases (15%). Differences between the cases and non-cases were not found with regard to out-patient visits.

Looking at the full range of primary and secondary services received by day centre visitors in the past year, it can be seen that secondary care had been received by a higher proportion of cases (65%) compared with non-cases (42%). The same trend was found among nightshelter residents but was even more pronounced among the day centre population. Only 13% of cases in day centres had received no services, compared with 35% of non-cases. *(Tables 8.17 and 8.18)*

As in nightshelters, 18% of the day centre population reported having a key worker and 2% did not know whether they had one. Twenty per cent of cases and 14% of non-cases had a key worker. Three per cent of day centre visitors had a care manager and 2% did not know (data not shown).

Treatment

Almost a third of those visiting day centres (31%) had received some form of psychiatric treatment; 47% of cases and 11% of non-cases. The proportion of non-cases receiving treatment was similar to that found in the nightshelter population, however a higher proportion of cases in day centres were receiving treatment compared with nightshelter cases (31%). This was due to the differential use of CNS drugs, rather than counselling or therapy. Anxiolytics were the most widely used medication among day centre cases - 17% were having these, while 10% were using each of hypnotics and analgesics. None of the non-cases were taking hypnotics and anxiolytics, however 3% were taking antidepressants, the same proportion as found among the cases. Counselling or therapy was being received by 13% of cases and 5% of non-cases, proportions similar to those among the nightshelter population. *(Table 8.19)*

8.7 Economic activity and finances

Economic activity

Over half of those interviewed in day centres were economically inactive (58%), with no difference between the cases and the non-cases, although within the economically inactive

123

category a larger proportion of the cases were permanently unable to work (28% compared with 19% of the non-cases). A third of day centre visitors were unemployed and 8% were working. Compared with the nightshelter residents, those sleeping rough were more likely to be economically inactive and less likely to be unemployed.

Respondents who were not working, but were not retired, were asked why they were not working; 27% of cases and 12% of non-cases said that the way they were feeling made work impossible; 30% and 22% respectively said a physical health problem made work impossible and for 24% of cases and 31% of non-cases, their current housing circumstances made it impossible to keep a paid job. *(Table 8.21)*

Finances

Sixty eight per cent of homeless people sleeping rough using day centres were receiving state benefits. There was no notable difference between the cases and non-cases. Income Support was the most widely received benefit, going to 58% of the day centre visitors (compared with 68% of nightshelter residents). Sickness Benefit was received by 15% of this population, a higher proportion than in any of the other samples, and Invalidity Pension was

received by 8%. A wide range of other benefits were received by between 1%-4% of homeless people sleeping rough. Sickness benefit was the only one to vary by GHQ12 score; 23% of cases were receiving this benefit compared with 5% of non-cases. *(Table 8.22)*

Sixty per cent of those using day centres had no source of income other than state benefits (56% of cases and 65% of non-cases). Nine per cent of those interviewed in day centres had another source of income in addition to state benefits while nearly a quarter of the sample reported receiving neither state benefits nor other sources of income. The median weekly income was £40-£59 a week among both cases and non-cases, the same as in nightshelters. *(Tables 8.23 and 8.24)*

As in nightshelters, no data were collected about social functioning or about stressful life events experienced over the last 6 months.

Notes and references

1.   The prevalence and socio-demographic sections are based on all respondents; subsequent sections comparing cases and non-cases exclude the few known cases of psychosis.

Table 8.1 Prevalence of alcohol dependence*

Homeless adults sleeping rough using day centres

Number of affirmative responses to the 12 alcohol dependence questions**	Percentage	Cumulative percentage
12	11	11
11	11	22
10	4	26
9	3	29
8	3	32
7	3	36
6	1	37
5	7	44
4	5	48
3	2	50
2	2	52
1	3	55
0	45	100
Base	*181*	*181*

* A score of 3 or more = alcohol dependence

A score of 7 or more = severe alcohol dependence

** See appendix B

Table 8.2 Prevalence of drug dependence

Homeless adults sleeping rough using day centres

Category of drug	Percentage
Dependence on ...*	
Cannabis	18
Stimulants	5
Hypnotics	4
Hallucinogens inc Ecstasy	4
Other drugs (heroin, opium)	7
Dependent on cannabis only	12
Dependent on cannabis & other drug	7
Dependent on non-cannabinoids	6
Dependent on any drug	**24**
Base	*181*

* Adults were defined as dependent on a drug if they had taken it every day for two weeks or more in the past year, and they had taken the drug more than prescribed, without prescription or to get high. Informants could be dependent on more than one drug.

Table 8.3 Socio-demographic characteristics by GHQ12 score

Homeless adults sleeping rough using day centres

	GHQ12 score		All
	4 or more	0-3	
	%	%	%
Sex			
Women	18	5	12
Men	82	95	88
Age			
16-24	22	14	19
25-34	34	28	31
35-44	18	24	20
45-54	19	22	20
55-64	8	11	9
Ethnicity			
White	98	98	98
West Indian/ African	2	-	1
Asian/ Oriental	-	-	-
Other	1	2	1
Marital status			
Married	1	5	2
Cohabiting	1	3	2
Single	57	73	64
Widowed	4	1	3
Divorced/ separated	38	19	30
Qualifications			
A level or higher	10	18	13
GCSE/ O level	16	16	16
Other	9	15	11
None	65	51	59
Employment status			
Working full-time	4	2	3
Working part-time	7	2	5
Unemployed	43	42	42
Economically inactive	46	55	50
Base	*103*	*78*	*181*

Table 8.4   Socio-demographic characteristics of adults with alcohol and drug dependence

Homeless adults sleeping rough using day centres

	Alcohol dependent (severe)	Drug dependent	Neither alcohol nor drug dependent	All
	%	%	%	%
Sex				
Men	93	90	84	12
Women	7	10	16	88
Age				
16-24	8	36	18	19
25-34	37	54	24	31
35-44	20	7	25	20
45-54	23	3	23	20
55-64	11	-	11	9
Ethnicity				
White	100	98	96	98
West Indian/ African	-	2	1	1
Asian/ Oriental	-	-	-	-
Other	-	-	2	1
Marital status				
Married	-	4	2	2
Cohabiting	1	4	2	2
Single	53	71	67	64
Widowed	4	3	2	3
Divorced/ separated	41	18	28	30
Qualifications				
A level or higher	10	11	17	13
GCSE/ O level	10	18	20	16
Other	7	14	11	11
None	73	58	52	59
Employment status				
Working full-time	5	4	1	3
Working part-time	5	5	6	5
Unemployed	30	41	48	42
Economically inactive	60	50	45	50
Base	*65*	*44*	*94*	*181*

Table 8.5   Alcohol drinking status by GHQ12 score

Homeless adults sleeping rough using day centres

| | GHQ12 score | | All |
| | 4 or more | 0-3 | |
	%	%	%
Current drinker*	80	85	82
Ex - drinker	13 ⎤ 16	11 ⎤ 15	12 ⎤ 15
Always non - drinker	3 ⎦	4 ⎦	3 ⎦
Don't know	4	-	3
Base	*101*	*77*	*178*

* Includes those who drink only very occasionally

Table 8.6   Alcohol consumption level by GHQ12 score

Homeless adults sleeping rough using day centres

| Alcohol consumption level | GHQ12 score | | All |
| | 4 or more | 0-3 | |
	%	%	%
Abstainer*	16 ⎤ 25	15 ⎤ 21	16 ⎤ 23
Occasional drinker	8 ⎦	6 ⎦	7 ⎦
Light	6	20	12
Moderate	9	13	11
Fairly heavy	7 ⎤	8 ⎤	8 ⎤
Heavy	6 ⎥ 60	6 ⎥ 46	6 ⎥ 54
Very heavy	47 ⎦	32 ⎦	41 ⎦
Base	*101*	*77*	*178*

* Includes informants who had not had an alcoholic drink in the past twelve months

Table 8.7   Symptoms of alcohol dependence by GHQ12 score

Homeless adults sleeping rough using day centres

| Symptoms reported | GHQ12 score | | All |
| | 4 or more | 0-3 | |
	Percentage experiencing symptom		
Skipped meals	52	38	45
Woke up next day unable to remember what done while drinking	51	38	45
Once started drinking, difficult to stop before became completely drunk	47	32	40
Stayed drunk for several days	44	32	39
Woke sweating due to drinking	44	32	39
Kept on drinking after promised myself not to	43	34	39
Deliberately tried to cut down/ stop but unable	43	26	36
Had strong drink in morning to get over effects of previous night's drinking	43	28	37
Often had alcoholic drink first thing in morning	42	34	38
Needed drink so badly, thought of nothing else	41	17	30
Hands shook a lot	39	23	32
Need more alcohol than used to for same effect	31	21	27
Any of above	**57**	**54**	**56**
Alcohol dependence*	54	46	51
Severe alcohol dependence**	46	23	36
Base	*101*	*77*	*178*

* 3 or more symptoms
** 7 or more symptoms

127

Table 8.8 Symptoms of alcohol dependence: symptomatic behaviour, loss of control and binge drinking by GHQ12 score

Homeless adults sleeping rough using day centres

Symptom and score	GHQ12 score		All
	4 or more	0 - 3	
	%	%	%
Binge drinking			
0	56	68	61
1	44	32	39
Symptomatic behaviour			
0	43	46	44
1	3	11	6
2	2	6	4
3	6	7	6
4	5	8	7
5	8 ⎱ 54	5 ⎱ 43	6 ⎱ 49
6	15	6	11
7	18	11	15
Loss of control			
0	46	54	50
1	3	17	9
2	8	7	7
3	16 ⎱ 51	10 ⎱ 29	13 ⎱ 41
4	27	12	21
Base	*101*	*77*	*178*

Table 8.9 Use of drugs by GHQ12 score

Homeless adults sleeping rough using day centres

Drug(s) taken	GHQ12 score		All
	4 or more	0-3	
	*Percentage using each drug**		
Cannabis	**31**	**31**	**31**
Stimulants	**13**	**18**	**15**
Amphetamines	11	14	12
Cocaine/crack	8	7	8
Hallucinogens inc. Ecstasy	**13**	**14**	**13**
Hallucinogens/ psychedelics	13	11	12
Ecstasy	11	7	9
Hypnotics	**17**	**11**	**14**
Sleeping tablets	14	6	10
Tranquilisers	14	10	12
Opiates	**18**	**8**	**13**
Heroin	12	5	9
Other opiates including methadone	11	6	9
Solvents	**2**	**4**	**3**
Any drug	**38**	**35**	**37**
Base	*101*	*77*	*178*

* Users had taken the drug more than prescribed, without prescription or to get high. They had used the drug in the past year, and more than five times in their lifetime. Informants may have taken more than one type of drug.

Table 8.10 Drug dependence (as measured by regularity of use) by GHQ12 score

Homeless adults sleeping rough using day centres

Drug(s) dependent on	GHQ12 score		All
	4 or more	0-3	
	*Percentage with drug dependence**		
Cannabis	19	18	18
Stimulants	4	6	6
Amphetamines	2	0	1
Cocaine/crack	3	5	4
Hallucinogens inc. Ecstasy	5	2	4
Hallucinogens/ psychedelics	5	2	4
Ecstasy	3	1	2
Hypnotics	6	2	4
Sleeping tablets	5	2	4
Tranquilisers	4	2	3
Opiates	8	4	7
Heroin	8	4	6
Other opiates including methadone	6	2	4
Solvents	1	0	0
Any non-cannabinoid drug	14	8	12
Any drug	25	22	24
Base	*101*	*77*	*178*

* Adults were defined as dependent on a drug if they had taken it every day for two weeks or more in the past year, and they had taken the drug more than prescribed, without prescription or to get high. Informants could be dependent on more than one drug.

Table 8.11 Cigarette smoking by GHQ12 score

Homeless adults sleeping rough using day centres

Cigarette smoking	GHQ12 score		All
	4 or more	0-3	
	%	%	%
Non-smoker	2	5	3
Ex-smoker	6	7	6
Light smoker	20 ⎤	12 ⎤	17 ⎤
Moderate smoker	28 ⎟ 92	26 ⎟ 88	27 ⎟ 90
Heavy smoker	44 ⎦	50 ⎦	46 ⎦
Base	*98*	*74*	*173*

Table 8.12 Self reported physical and mental long-standing illness by GHQ12 score

Homeless adults sleeping rough using day centres

	GHQ12 score		All
	4 or more	0 - 3	
	%	%	%
Physical illness only	38	41	39
Physical and mental illness	20	8	14
Mental illness only	10	3	7
No long-standing illness	32	48	39
Base	*101*	*77*	*178*

129

Table 8.13 Long-standing physical complaints by GHQ12 score

Homeless adults sleeping rough using day centres

Physical complaint	GHQ12 score		All
	4 or more	0-3	
	Percentage with each complaint		
Respiratory system complaints	**23**	**14**	**19**
Bronchitis/emphysema	6	4	5
Asthma	16	4	11
Hayfever	-	-	-
Other respiratory complaints	5	6	6
Musculo-skeletal complaints	**19**	**16**	**18**
Arthritis/rheumatism/ fibrositis	4	8	6
Back & neck problems/ slipped disk	4	2	3
Other problems of bones/ joints/muscles	13	6	10
Nervous system complaints	**12**	**5**	**9**
Epilepsy	8	3	6
Migraine	-	3	1
Other nervous system complaints	5	-	3
Digestive system complaints	**11**	**8**	**9**
Stomach complaints & ulcers	5	5	5
Large & small intestine complaints	-	3	1
Other digestive complaints	5	-	3
Heart/ circulation complaints	**4**	**4**	**4**
Stroke and heart complaints	3	4	4
Blood pressure complaints	1	-	1
Blood vessel complaints	-	0	0
Skin complaints	**2**	**5**	**3**
Genito-urinary system complaints	**4**	**-**	**2**
Endocrine disorders	**2**	**3**	**2**
Neoplasms (and benign lumps or cysts)	**1**	**4**	**2**
Eye complaints	**2**	**1**	**1**
Infectious and parasitic diseases	**0**	**-**	**0**
Ear complaints	**0**	**-**	**0**
Blood disorders	**-**	**-**	**-**
Any physical complaint	**57**	**49**	**54**
Base	*101*	*77*	*178*

Table 8.14 Access to a doctor by GHQ12 score

Homeless adults sleeping rough using day centres

Access to a doctor	GHQ12 score		All
	4 or more	0-3	
	%	*%*	*%*
If feeling unwell is there a doctor or medical centre you could go to?			
yes	75	82	78
no	24	17	21
don't know	1	1	1
Registered with a doctor?			
yes	66	48	58
no	33	50	41
don't know	1	3	2
Base	*101*	*77*	*178*

Table 8.15   GP consultations by GHQ12 score

Homeless adults sleeping rough using day centres

Type of consultation		GHQ12 score		All
		4 or more	0-3	
		Percentage consulting GP*		
Consulted GP in past 2 weeks for physical complaint(s) only		22	14	18
Consulted GP in past 2 weeks for mental complaint(s) only		10	1	6
Consulted GP in past 2 weeks for physical and mental complaint(s) together		4	2	3
Consulted GP in past 2 weeks for any reason		35	16	27
		%	*%*	*%*
Whether consulted GP in past 12 months for physical complaint	Yes	72	52	64
	No	23	44	32
	Unknown	5	4	4
Whether consulted GP in past 12 months for mental complaint	Yes	47	14	33
	No	48	82	63
	Unknown	5	4	4
Whether consulted GP in past 12 months for any complaint	Yes	80	53	68
	No	20	47	32
	Unknown	0	0	0
Base		*101*	*77*	*178*

* Consultations refer to those made on the informant's own behalf and informants may have had more than one consultation

Table 8.16   Location of GP consultation

Homeless adults sleeping rough using day centres who spoke to a doctor on their own behalf in the past 2 weeks

Doctor contacted at:	
	Percentage speaking with doctor at each location*
GP surgery/ health centre	72%
Day centre/ hostel clinic	20%
Spoke to GP on telephone	4%
Other	4%
Base	*48*

*   Percentages could total more than 100% as people may have contacted a doctor on more than one occasion, at different locations

Table 8.17   Percentage of people who had been in-patients or out-patients in the past year and reason for hospital stay or visit by GHQ12 score

Homeless adults sleeping rough using day centres

	In-patient stay			Out-patient visit		
	GHQ12 score			GHQ12 score		
	4 or more	0-3	All	4 or more	0-3	All
	%	%	%	%	%	%
Physical problem(s)	38	11	26	31	33	32
Mental problem(s)	2 ⎫ 45	3 ⎫ 15	3 ⎫ 32	2 ⎫ 39	1 ⎫ 38	1 ⎫ 38
Both physical & mental problem(s)*	6 ⎭	1 ⎭	4 ⎭	6 ⎭	4 ⎭	5 ⎭
No such stay or visit	55	85	68	61	62	62
Base	101	77	178	101	77	178

*   includes more than one stay or visit for different problems, or one stay or visit for both types of problem

Table 8.18   Profile of GP use, in-patient stays and out-patient visits during the past year by GHQ12 score

Homeless adults sleeping rough using day centres

Services received	GHQ12 score		All
	4 or more	0 - 3	
	%	%	%
None	13	35	23
GP only	22	23	22
GP and out-patient visit	18	18	18
GP and in-patient stay	24	3	15
GP and in-patient stay & out-patient visit	15 65	9 42	13 55
Out-patient visit only	1	9	4
Out-patient visit & in-patient stay	4	1	3
In-patient stay only	2	2	2
Base	101	77	178

Where data on in-patient stays and out-patient visits were missing,

respondents are categorised with regard only to GP use

Table 8.19 Proportion of people taking each type of CNS medication and having counselling or therapy by GHQ12 score

Homeless adults sleeping rough using day centres

Type of medication or therapy	GHQ12 score		All
	4 or more	0-3	
	Percentage having medication or receiving therapy		
Hypnotics and anxiolytics	**21**	**1**	**12**
Hypnotics	10	1	6
Anxiolytics	17	0	10
Analgesics	**10**	**0**	**6**
Antiepileptics	**6**	**3**	**5**
Drugs used in treatment of substance dependence	**5**	**1**	**3**
Antidepressant drugs	**3**	**3**	**3**
Tricyclic antidepressants	1	3	2
Serotonin reuptake inhibitors	2	0	1
Anticholinergic drugs	**1**	**0**	**1**
Any CNS drugs	**38**	**8**	**25**
Any counselling or therapy	**13**	**5**	**9**
Any psychiatric treatment, medication or therapy	**47**	**11**	**31**
Base	*101*	*77*	*178*

Table 8.20 Economic activity in the past 7 days by GHQ12 score

Homeless adults sleeping rough using day centres

	GHQ12 score		All	
	4 or more	0-3		
	%	%	%	
Employed				
Employed - at work	11	4	8	
Unemployed				
Looking for work	30	37	33	
Waiting to start job		31	38	34
already obtained	1	1	1	
Economically inactive				
Intending to look, temporarily sick	12	4	9	
Permanently unable to work	28	58	19 58	24 58
Retired	1	3	2	
Full time education	-	3	2	
Other	17	29	22	
Base	*101*	*77*	*178*	

Table 8.21 Reasons for not working by GHQ12 score

Homeless adults sleeping rough using day centres who were not working, but were not retired

Why not working?	GHQ12 score		All
	4 or more	0-3	
	%	%	%
Way feeling makes work impossible	27	12	20
Physical health problem makes work impossible	30	22	26
Current housing circumstances make it impossible to keep a paid job	24	31	27
Have not found suitable paid job	13	25	18
Do not want/ need paid job	6	10	8
Base	*84*	*71*	*155*

133

Table 8.22   Receipt of State Benefits by GHQ12 score

Homeless adults sleeping rough using day centres

Type of benefit	GHQ12 score		All
	4 or more	0-3	
	*Percentage receiving benefit**		
Income Support	56	60	58
Sickness Benefit	23	5	15
Invalidity pension, benefit or allowance	9	8	8
Disability Living Allowance	5	3	4
Severe Disablement Allowance	5	1	3
Unemployment Benefit	0	7	3
Old Age Pension	3	3	3
Mobility Allowance	4	0	2
Invalid Care Allowance	4	0	2
War widow's pension	2	0	1
Any other state pension	2	0	1
War Disablement pension	2	0	1
Industrial Disablement Allowance	2	0	1
Attendance Allowance	2	0	1
Disability Working Allowance	2	0	1
Maternity Allowance	2	0	1
Other	4	4	4
Any State Benefit	**67**	**71**	**68**
Base	*101*	*77*	*178*

*   Figures for specific benefits represent the minimum percentage receiving benefit as questions were not answered by 2% - 8% of adults.

Table 8.23   Receipt of State Benefits and other sources of income by GHQ12 score

Homeless adults sleeping rough using day centres

In receipt of:	GHQ12 score		All
	4 or more	0-3	
	%	*%*	*%*
State Benefits only; no other source of income	56	65	60
State Benefits and other source(s) of income*	11	6	9
No State Benefits; other source(s) of income only	10	6	8
No State Benefits or other source of income	23	24	23
Base	*101*	*77*	*178*

*   Respondents were asked about receipt of earned income/salary, income from self-employment and income from any other source.

Table 8.24 Personal gross income by GHQ12 score

Homeless adults sleeping rough using day centres

Yearly income	Weekly income	GHQ12 score		All
		4 or more	0-3	
		%	%	%
No income		**17**	**15**	**16**
Less than £1000	Less than £20	1	0	0
£1000 - £1999	£20 - £39	14	7	11
£2000 - £2999	£40 - £59	34 ⎤	43 ⎤	38 ⎤
£3000 - £3999	£60 - £79	22 ⎥ 72	27 ⎥ 82	24 ⎥ 76
£4000 - £4999	£80 - £99	- ⎦	5 ⎦	2 ⎦
£5000 - £5999	£100 - £119	1 ⎤	- ⎤	0 ⎤
£6000 - £6999	£120 - £139	- ⎥	- ⎥	- ⎥
£7000 - £7999	£140 - £159	- ⎥ 6	- ⎥ 1	0 ⎥ 4
£8000 - £8999	£160 - £179	4 ⎥	- ⎥	2 ⎥
£9000 - £9999	£180 - £199	2 ⎦	- ⎦	1 ⎦
£10000 - £10999	£200 - £219	- ⎤	- ⎤	- ⎤
£11000 - £11999	£220 - £239	0 ⎥	- ⎥	- ⎥
£12000 - £12999	£240 - £259	- ⎥ 0	- ⎥ -	- ⎥ 0
£13000 - £13999	£260 - £279	- ⎥	- ⎥	- ⎥
£14000 - £14999	£280 - £299	- ⎦	- ⎦	- ⎦
£15000 or more	£300 or more	1	2	1
Don't know		**5**	**1**	**3**
Median weekly income		£40 - £59	£40 - £59	£40 - £59
Base		*101*	*77*	*178*

Appendix A   Non-response and weighting

Part A1 of this appendix discusses the issue of non-response and examines the reasons why selected informants refused. The second part outlines the issues that were considered for each sample in weighting the data for disproportionate sampling and non-response and details how the weighting was carried out.

A1.   Non-response

Introduction

On this survey where very little is known about the target population, the only information which can be used to compare survey responders with non-responders is that which has been specifically collected for this purpose. Wherever possible interviewers identified whether non-responding adults were eligible for the survey according to the criteria of their respective samples, and found out their age and sex, and in PSLA, their household size.

Collecting information to examine topic related non-response, such as details of mental state or the extent of intoxication, was more difficult and was not attempted in a standardised way; in order to make meaningful comparisons between responders and non-responders, interviewers would have to make assessments of the whole sample using consistent rules, sometimes in less than half a minute. However, some illumination on possible non-response bias can be gained by examining the reasons given by non-responders, which interviewers recorded wherever possible. It should be noted that bases were small and that the reasons given by informants may not be reliable. Also, in nightshelters and day centres, interviewers noted their observations of the mental state of non-responders, including reasons why staff may have advised them against interviewing a particular subject.

Reasons for non-response

Just as in the survey in private households, apathy was the most common reason given by respondents for refusal; between 20% (in PSLA) and 44% (in hostels) said they could not be bothered, as did 36% of the refusers in the private household survey. The proportion of adults reporting sickness or personal problems as a reason for not taking part was highest in hostels (36%), nightshelters (29%) and day centres (26%) and lowest in PSLA (14%). By comparison, only 4% of refusers in the survey in private households cited sickness and 11% cited personal problems. Although it appears that a large proportion of refusers on this survey were in poor physical or mental health, it is not clear whether those who were ill were more likely to refuse. Indeed, among adults who responded to the survey, the proportion who reported poor health, any physical or mental problem, or alcohol or drug dependence, was also highest in hostels (71%), nightshelters (83%) and day centres (76%) and lowest in PSLA (56%).

In nightshelters, of the 33 who refused the survey, interviewers felt it was relevant to make notes on 13 selected informants in addition to the reasons they gave for refusing. Of these, 6 were drunk, 4 had mental health problems, 2 were high on drugs and 1 had alcohol problems. In day centres, of the 51 who refused the survey, interviewers noted that 3 were drunk and 3 were suffering from mental health problems or stress. In total, interviewers withdrew from 16 interviews, mostly on the advice of staff before attempting any interviewing, because of the potential danger to themselves or the danger of causing distress to the informant: 3 were in hostels, 7 in nightshelters and 6 were in day centres.

Further analysis of non-response was carried out after weighting for unequal chances of selection. This is covered in the weighting section.

A2.   Weighting

Introduction

In any sample whose elements have been chosen with unequal probabilities, unbiased estimation of population quantities requires the use of compensating weights which are inversely proportional to the selection probabilities.[1] Only the relative sizes of these weights are important, not the gross magnitude. However, it is convenient to scale the weights so that the weighted sample size is similar to the actual sample size. Through scaling, the weighted sample size in some way reflects the actual sample size as an indicator of its precision.

Having weighted the data for unequal chances of selection, it can be examined for signs of bias arising from non-response. Weighting for differential non-response according to region was not considered for this survey, as response rates would have been based on small sample sizes and the figures are likely to have been unreliable.

Where there are apparent differences with respect to some survey variable between adults who responded and those who did not, small sample sizes may not allow us to identify a statistically significant bias. If certain population subgroups are found to be significantly under-represented due to non-response bias, compensating weights can be applied to responding adults in those subgroups. At the last stage, scaling takes place to ensure the weighted sample size is the same as the actual sample size.

The usual effect of weighting is to increase sampling errors and thereby reduce the effective sample size. It is possible to estimate the effective sample size of a weighted sample, that is, the size of an equal probability sample with the same precision.

Weighting the hostels sample

Weighting was considered for the following aspects of the sample design and response:

Unequal probabilities of selection

There are two reasons why this was not an equal probability sample:

(i)   Quotas were allocated to regions based on the numbers of statutory homeless households in hostels, and then allocated among the 363 local authorities which responded to our request for information. Having obtained more reliable estimates of the population size from the hostels in selected local authorities, quotas were re-allocated within these areas but this did not compensate for all the change found. Hence further compensation was required at the local authority level using a weighting factor, f_0 equal to f_2/f_1:

$$f_1 = \frac{\textit{revised estimate of population size}}{\substack{\textit{number of statutory homeless} \\ \textit{households in hostels}}}$$

$$f_2 = \frac{\textit{number of quotas after reallocation}}{\textit{initial number of sample quotas}}$$

(ii)   Individuals within each local authority also had an uneven chance of selection which was based on the sampling fraction of hostels drawn from those in the area, f_3, and the sampling interval applied to residents within each hostel, f_4.

The overall effect of these uneven chances of selection was measured as the product of the three factors:

$$f_0 \times f_3 \times f_4$$

and the compensating weight was the reciprocal of this.

Substitution

Hostels which were ineligible or refused to take part were substituted by another hostel. No substitution was made for individuals. Since reserve addresses were selected at the same time as the original sample, substitute hostels had the same chance of selection as the refusing hostel.[2] The selection probabilities of hostels which were used to substitute ineligible addresses are based on the ineligibility rate in the original sample of hostels. Because relatively small numbers of hostels were sampled in any one local authority, estimates of the variability in eligibility rates between local authorities cannot be estimated with reliability. However, it is reasonable to assume that the ineligibility rate will not differ systematically between authorities since a number of eligibility checks had been made on every hostel before sampling. There was consequently no weighting for substitution.

Relative size of the weights

Having weighted for unequal probabilities of selection, a small proportion of the sample were found to have very high weights (up to 7). The increase in sample variance arising from giving such weights to a small part of the sample was considered intolerable yet if the weights were trimmed, some bias would be incurred.[3] After an investigation, it was apparent that these high weights involved residents in large hostels in three local authorities where only a small proporiton of residents had been sampled, and the ratio of the sizes of the non-statutory and statutory homeless population in hostels was high. In all three authorities, there were other quotas sampled and the weights within these were of a reasonable size. Under the assumption that adults in other hostels in the same local authorities were broadly similar to those with the high weights, it was possible to trim the high weights yet minimise the possibility of bias. This was achieved by increasing the weights in each of the three local authorities by such a proportion as to compensate for the lower chances of selection of residents in the affected hostels. In this way the highest weight was set to 4.

Non-response

After weighting for disproportionate chances of selection, information on the age and sex of adults who co-operated with the survey were compared with those who refused and those who could not be contacted, for instance because they did not stay long at the hostel. There was a disproportionably high refusal rate among men; while 67% of respondents were men, they made up 91% of the refusers. Hence men were under-represented in the survey and were given a compensatory weight:

$$W_0 = \frac{number\ of\ men\ interviewed + number\ of\ men\ refusing}{number\ of\ men\ interviewed}$$

Scaling

Finally a scaling factor was applied to all weights so the weighted sample size was the same as the actual sample size: 530.

Sample efficiency

An approximate estimate of the efficiency of the weighted sample compared with a simple random sample is 71%. Another way of expressing this is that the effective sample size was 375 even though 530 interviews were collected.

Weighting the PSLA sample

Weighting was considered for the following aspects of the sample design and response:

Incomplete response from the local authority housing departments

Local authorities which did not return information about PSLA had no chance of selection. However, official statistics on the number of households temporarily placed by local authorities in PSLA were found to be approximately in proportion with the counts obtained directly from the responding local authorities in which addresses did have a chance of selection. Hence the sample of addresses was approximately self-weighting.

Under-sampling of multi-household addresses

The majority of PSL addresses contained only one household. Where more than one was present, interviewers were instructed to interview at up to two of them. At addresses with more than two households, this meant taking a subsample of households using pre-assigned sampling numbers. In such instances, respondents were assigned weights equal to the number of households found divided by the number which were selected.

Substitution for ineligible addresses

If an address in the original sample was found to be ineligible, most commonly because it was empty at the time, interviewers attempted to interview at the designated substitute address. The chances that a reserve address might be selected was therefore determined by the local ineligibility rate. Since PSLA addresses in some local authorities were more likely to be ineligible than in others, weights were applied which corresponded to the eligibility rate in each authority. The eligibility rate was based on the outcome of calls on addresses in the original sample, that is, excluding reserves:

$$eligibility\ rate = \frac{number\ of\ eligible\ addresses\ in\ the\ LA}{number\ of\ addresses\ selected\ in\ the\ LA}$$

Selecting one person per household

Because only one of the adults in the eligible age-range was interviewed, adults who lived in large households had a lower chance of inclusion in the survey. Compensatory weights were applied to respondents from large households equivalent to the number of eligible people in their household.

Non-response

Although it may have been desirable to look at regional response rates, such as those for Greater London compared with elsewhere, these would have been based on small bases and figures would have been unreliable.

A comparison of responders with non-responders showed little apparent difference according to household size or the ages of selected informants, and none of the differences were found to be statistically significant. Hence no non-response weighting was carried out.

Scaling

The weights were adjusted by a scaling factor which brought the weighted sample size to 268: the size of the actual sample.

Sample efficiency

The efficiency of the weighted sample was approximately 70% compared with a simple random sample. The precision gained from this sample design with 268 informants is of broadly similar magnitude to that of a simple random sample of about 187 informants.

Weighting the nightshelters sample

The following factors were considered in weighting the sample in nightshelters:

The exclusion of nightshelters with less than an average of 5 residents aged 16 to 64 per night

Such nightshelters were not sampled as it would not have been cost effective to sample and interview there. However, it is assumed that the characteristics of the residents aged 16 to 64 in these nightshelters are the same as those of the nightshelter residents who were surveyed.

Sub-sampling of smaller nightshelters

Only half the nightshelters with less than an average of 10 eligible residents per night were

139

sampled, and a compensatory weight of 2 was given for respondents in these.

Substitutions

Two reserve nightshelters were contacted. In both cases, the original sampled nightshelter which dropped out had been selected with a probability of one, so no weighting was required.

Sampling within the nightshelter

The sampling fraction within nightshelters varied between one in every four residents, and every resident. To compensate for this, the weight was multiplied by the reciprocal of the sampling fraction.

Frequency of use

Because adults who stayed in nightshelters regularly were more likely to have been picked up in the survey, it was important to obtain a measure of their frequency of nightshelter use. All adults who were selected for interview were asked how many nights they had stayed in any nightshelter in the previous seven nights. Although their answers reflected their use of nightshelters only at a point in time, they were used to broadly group nightshelter residents into 'infrequent visitors' and 'regulars' depending on whether they had stayed in a nightshelter on 3 or more nights a week. The average number of nights stayed by an infrequent visitor in the previous seven nights was 1.4, compared with 6.4 for regular visitors. The weighting factor to compensate for different frequencies of use was the reciprocal of the average number of nights spent in nightshelters.

Where respondents did not answer the question on frequency of nightshelter use, they were given a weight corresponding to the overall average number of nights spent in nightshelters (5.5).

Non-response

Sample sizes of non-responders and responders were too small to allow an investigation of non-response.

Scaling

The weighted sample size was scaled down to 186, approximately equal to the actual sample size, by applying a scaling factor to all weights.

Sample efficiency

The weighted sample efficiency was approximately 67%, and the effective sample size was 122.

Weighting the day centres sample

The issues were identical to those in nightshelters, although it is worth mentioning that people who slept rough but did not use day centres had no chance of selection in this survey and since nothing is known about how they vary from the rough sleepers who were interviewed, it is not possible to make any weighting adjustments for this.

The exclusion of day centres with less than an average of 5 eligible visitors

As for nightshelters.

Sub-sampling of smaller day centres

Only half the day centres with less than an average of 40 eligible visitors a day were sampled and a compensatory weight of 2 was given for respondents in these.

Substitutions

Seven reserve day centres were contacted. Those that were substituted in place of smaller day centres (size 40 or less) were given a weight of 2 to compensate for the lower chance of selection of day centres of this size.

Sampling within the day centre

The sampling fraction applied to eligible visitors in day centres varied between 1 in 3 and 1 in 1. To compensate for this, the weight was multiplied by the reciprocal of the sampling fraction.

Frequency of use

Just as in nightshelters, day centre visitors who were selected for interview were asked the number of days in the past week they visited a day centre. Their replies were used to group them broadly into 'infrequent visitors' and 'regulars'. Infrequent visitors who attended a day centre on less than 3 days in the previous week were found to have attended on 1.4 days on average in contrast with regular attenders for whom the average was 4.9 days attendance. For the few who did not answer this question, it was assumed they visited on about 4 days which was the average number of days overall.

To compensate for over-representing regular visitors, a weight was applied equivalent to the reciprocal of the average number of days in attendance at any day centre.

Non-response

Sample sizes of non-responders and responders were too small to allow an investigation of non-response.

Scaling

The weighted sample size was scaled down to 181, which was the actual sample size, by applying a scaling factor to all weights.

Sample efficiency

The weighted sample efficiency was approximately 76%, and the effective sample size was 139.

References

1. Elliot, D; (1991) *Weighting for non-response. A survey researcher's guide*, OPCS London

2. Elliot, D; (1993) The use of substitution in sampling, *Survey Methodology Bulletin* no. 33, OPCS London

3. Kish, L; (1992), Weighting for unequal P_i, *Journal of Official Statistics*, Vol 8, No. 2, pp.183-200 Statistics Sweden

Appendix B Measurement of psychiatric disorders

B.1 Calculation of CIS-R symptom scores

Fatigue

Scores relate to fatigue or feeling tired or lacking in energy in the past week.
Score one for each of:
- Symptom present on four days or more
- Symptom present for more than three hours in total on any day
- Subject had to push him/herself to get things done on at least one occasion
- Symptom present when subject doing things he/she enjoys or used to enjoy at least once

Sleep problems

Scores relate to problems with getting to sleep, or otherwise, with sleeping more than is usual for the subject in the past week.
Score one for each of:
- Had problems with sleep for four nights or more
- Spent at least 4 hours trying to get to sleep on the night with least sleep
- Spent at least 1 hour trying to get to sleep on the night with least sleep
- Spent three hours or more trying to get to sleep on four nights or more
- Slept for at least 4 hours longer than usual for subject on any night
- Slept for at least 1 hour longer than usual for subject on any night
- Slept for more than three hours longer than usual for subject on four nights or more

Irritability

Scores relate to feelings of irritability, being short-tempered or angry in the past week.
Score one for each of:
- Symptom present for four days or more
- Symptom present for more than one hour on any day
- Wanted to shout at someone (even if subject had not actually shouted)
- Had arguments, rows or quarrels or lost temper with someone and felt it was unjustified on at least one occasion

Worry

Scores relate to subject's experience of worry in the past week, other than worry about physical health.
Score one for each of:
- Symptom present on four or more days
- Has been worrying too much in view of circumstances
- Symptom has been very unpleasant
- Symptom lasted over three hours in total on any day

Depression

Applies to subjects who felt sad, miserable or depressed or unable to enjoy or take an interest in things as much as usual, in the past week. Scores relate to the subject's experience in the past week.
Score one for each of:
- Unable to enjoy or take an interest in things as much as usual
- Symptom present on four days or more
- Symptom lasted for more than three hours in total on any day
- When sad, miserable or depressed subject did not become happier when something nice happened, or when in company

Depressive ideas

Applies to subjects who had a score of 1 for depression. Scores relate to experience in the past week.
Score one for each of:
- Felt guilty or blamed him/herself at least once when things went wrong when it had not been his/her fault
- Felt not as good as other people
- Felt hopeless
- Felt that life isn't worth living
- Thought of killing him/herself

Anxiety
Scores relate to feeling generally anxious, nervous or tense in the past week. These feelings were not the result of a phobia.
Score one for each of:
- Symptom present on four or more days
- Symptom had been very unpleasant
- When anxious, nervous or tense, had one or more of following symptoms:
  heart racing or pounding
  hands sweating or shaking
  feeling dizzy
  difficulty getting breath
  butterflies in stomach
  dry mouth
  nausea or feeling as though he/she wanted to vomit
- Symptom present for more than three hours in total on any one day

Obsessions
Scores relate to the subject's experience of having repetitive unpleasant thoughts or ideas in the past week.
Score one for each of:
- Symptom present on four or more days
- Tried to stop thinking any of these thoughts
- Became upset or annoyed when had these thoughts
- Longest episode of the symptom was 1/4 hour or longer

Concentration and forgetfulness
Scores relate to the subject's experience of concentration problems and forgetfulness in the past week.
Score one for each of:
- Symptoms present for four days or more
- Could not always concentrate on a TV programme, read a newspaper article or talk to someone without mind wandering
- Problems with concentration stopped subject from getting on with things he/she used to do or would have liked to do
- Forgot something important

Somatic symptoms
Scores relate to the subject's experience in the past week of any ache, pain or discomfort which was brought on or made worse by feeling low,

anxious or stressed.
Score one for each of:
- Symptom present for four days or more
- Symptom lasted more than three hours on any day
- Symptom had been very unpleasant
- Symptom bothered subject when doing something interesting

Compulsions
Scores relate to the subject's experience of doing things over again when subject had already done them in the past week.
Score one for each of:
- Symptom present on four days or more
- Subject tried to stop repeating behaviour
- Symptom made subject upset or annoyed with him/herself
- Repeated behaviour three or more times when it had already been done

Phobias
Scores relate to subject's experience of phobias or avoidance in the past week
Score one for each of:
- Felt nervous/anxious about a situation or thing four or more times
- On occasions when felt anxious, nervous or tense, had one or more of following symptoms:
  heart racing or pounding
  hands sweating or shaking
  feeling dizzy
  difficulty getting breath
  butterflies in stomach
  dry mouth
  nausea or feeling as though he/she wanted to vomit
- Avoided situation or thing at least once because it would have made subject anxious, nervous or tense
- Avoided situation or thing four times or more because it would have made subject anxious, nervous or tense

Worry about physical health
Scores relate to experience of the symptom in the past week.
Score one for each of:
- Symptom present on four days or more

- Subject felt he/she had been worrying too much in view of actual health
- Symptom had been very unpleasant
- Subject could not be distracted by doing something else

Panic

Applies to subjects who felt anxious, nervous or tense in the past week and the scores relate to the resultant feelings of panic, or of collapsing and losing control in the past week.
Score one for each of:
- Symptom experienced once
- Symptom experienced more than once
- Symptom had been very unpleasant or unbearable
- An episode lasted longer than 10 minutes

B.2 Algorithms for production of ICD-10 diagnoses of neurosis from the CIS-R ('scores' refer to CIS-R scores)

F32.00 Mild depressive episode without somatic symptoms

1. Symptom duration ≥ 2 weeks

2. *Two or more from:*

   - depressed mood
   - loss of interest
   - fatigue

3. *Two or three from:*

   - reduced concentration
   - reduced self-esteem
   - ideas of guilt
   - pessimism about future
   - suicidal ideas or acts
   - disturbed sleep
   - diminished appetite

4. Social impairment

5. *Fewer than four from:*

   - lack of normal pleasure /interest
   - loss of normal emotional reactivity

- a.m. waking ≥ 2 hours early
- loss of libido
- diurnal variation in mood
- diminished appetite
- loss of ≥ 5% body weight
- psychomotor agitation
- psychomotor retardation

F32.01 Mild depressive episode with somatic symptoms

1. Symptom duration ≥ 2 weeks

2. *Two or more from:*

   - depressed mood
   - loss of interest
   - fatigue

3. *Two or three from:*

   - reduced concentration
   - reduced self-esteem
   - ideas of guilt
   - pessimism about future
   - suicidal ideas or acts
   - disturbed sleep
   - diminished appetite

4. Social impairment

5. *Four or more from:*

   - lack of normal pleasure /interest
   - loss of normal emotional reactivity
   - a.m. waking ≥ 2 hours early
   - loss of libido
   - diurnal variation in mood
   - diminished appetite
   - loss of 5% body weight
   - psychomotor agitation
   - psychomotor retardation

F32.10 Moderate depressive episode without somatic symptoms

1. Symptom duration ≥2 weeks

2. *Two or more from:*

   - depressed mood
   - loss of interest
   - fatigue

3. *Four or more* from:

- reduced concentration
- reduced self-esteem
- ideas of guilt
- pessimism about future
- suicidal ideas or acts
- disturbed sleep
- diminished appetite

4. Social impairment

5. *Fewer than four* from:

- lack of normal pleasure/interest
- loss of normal emotional reactivity
- a.m. waking ≥ 2 hours early
- loss of libido
- diurnal variation in mood
- diminished appetite
- loss of ≥ 5% body weight
- psychomotor agitation
- psychomotor retardation

F32.11 Moderate depressive episode with somatic symptoms

1. Symptom duration ≥2 weeks

2. *Two or more* from:

- depressed mood
- loss of interest
- fatigue

3. *Four or more* from:

- reduced concentration
- reduced self-esteem
- ideas of guilt
- pessimism about future
- suicidal ideas or acts
- disturbed sleep
- diminished appetite

4. Social impairment

5. *Four or more* from:

- lack of normal pleasure /interest
- loss of normal emotional reactivity

- a.m. waking ≥2 hours early
- loss of libido
- diurnal variation in mood
- diminished appetite
- loss of ≥ 5% body weight
- psychomotor agitation
- psychomotor retardation

F32.2 Severe depressive episode

1. *All three* from:

- depressed mood
- loss of interest
- fatigue

2. *Four or more* from:

- reduced concentration
- reduced self-esteem
- ideas of guilt
- pessimism about future
- suicidal ideas or acts
- disturbed sleep
- diminished appetite

3. Social impairment

4. *Four or more* from:

- lack of normal pleasure /interest
- loss of normal emotional reactivity
- a.m. waking ≥ 2 hours early
- loss of libido
- diurnal variation in mood
- diminished appetite
- loss of ≥ 5% body weight
- psychomotor agitation
- psychomotor retardation

F40.00 Agoraphobia without panic disorder

1. Fear of open spaces and related aspects: crowds, distance from home, travelling alone
2. Social impairment
3. Avoidant behaviour must be prominent feature
4. Overall phobia score ≥ 2
5. No panic attacks

F40.01 Agoraphobia with panic disorder

1. Fear of open spaces and related aspects: crowds, distance from home, travelling alone
2. Social impairment
3. Avoidant behaviour must be prominent feature
4. Overall phobia score ≥ 2
5. Panic disorder (overall panic score ≥ 2)

F40.1 Social phobias

1. Fear of scrutiny by other people: eating or speaking in public etc.
2. Social impairment
3. Avoidant behaviour must be prominent feature
4. Overall phobia score ≥ 2

F40.2 Specific (isolated) phobias

1. Fear of specific situations or things, e.g. animals, insects, heights, blood, flying, etc.
2. Social impairment
3. Avoidant behaviour must be prominent feature
4. Overall phobia score ≥ 2

F41.0 Panic disorder

1. Criteria for phobic disorders not met
2. Recent panic attacks
3. Anxiety-free between attacks
4. Overall panic score ≥ 2

F41.1 Generalised Anxiety Disorder

1. Duration ≥ 6 months
2. Free-floating anxiety
3. Autonomic overactivity
4. Overall anxiety score ≥ 2

F41.2 Mixed anxiety and depressive disorder

1. (Sum of scores for each CIS-R section) ≥ 12
2. Criteria for other categories not met

F42 Obsessive-Compulsive Disorder

1. Duration ≥ 2 weeks
2. At least one act/thought resisted
3. Social impairment
4. Overall scores:
   obsession score=4, or
   compulsion score=4, or
   obsession+compulsion scores ≥ 6

Hierarchical organisation of psychiatric disorders

The following rules (see Figure B.1) were used to allocate individuals who received more than one diagnosis of neurosis to the appropriate category.

Grouping neurotic and psychotic disorders into broad categories

The final step was to group some of the diagnoses into broad diagnostic categories prior to analysis.

Figure B1 Hierarchical organisation of psychiatric disorders

Disorder 1	Disorder 2	Priority
Depressive episode (any severity)	Phobia	Depressive episode (any severity)
Depressive episode (mild)	OCD	OCD
Depressive episode (moderate)	OCD	Depressive episode (moderate)
Depressive episode (severe)	OCD	Depressive episode (severe)
Depressive episode (mild)	Panic disorder	Panic disorder
Depressive episode (moderate)	Panic disorder	Depressive episode (moderate)
Depressive episode (any severity)	GAD	Depressive episode (any severity)
Phobia (any)	OCD	OCD
Agoraphobia	GAD	Agoraphobia
Social phobia	GAD	Social phobia
Specific phobia	GAD	GAD
Panic disorder	OCD	Panic disorder
OCD	GAD	OCD
Panic disorder	GAD	Panic disorder

GAD = Generalised Anxiety Disorder OCD = Obsessive– Compulsive Disorder

Depressive episode

F32.00 and F32.01 were grouped to produce mild depressive episode (i.e. with or without somatic symptoms). F32.10 and F32.11 were similarly grouped to produce moderate depressive episode. Mild depressive episode, moderate depressive episode and severe depressive episode (F32.2) were then combined to produce the final category of depressive episode.

Phobias

The ICD-10 phobic diagnoses F40.00, F40.01, F40.1 and F40.2, were combined into one category of phobia.

This produced six categories of neurosis for analysis:

> Mixed anxiety and depressive disorder
> Generalised Anxiety Disorder
> Depressive episode
> All phobias
> Obsessive Compulsive Disorder
> Panic disorder

B3. The GHQ12

This is reproduced in Appendix D, Survey Documents, Schedule GH. The overall score is calculated by attributing a score of 1 for the response "much more than usual" or " rather more than usual" to items where agreement indicates illness (negative items such as feeling constantly under strain). Similarly a score of 1 is ascribed for the response "more so than usual" or "same as usual" for items where agreement indicates health (positive items, such as enjoying day to day activities). The questionnaire is copyrighted "David Goldberg, 1978" and can only be used with the permission of The NFER-NELSON Publishing Company Ltd.

B4. Psychosis

Making assessments of psychotic rather than neurotic disorders is more problematic for lay interviewers. A structured questionnaire is too restrictive and a semi-structured questionnaire requires the use of clinical judgements. Therefore OPCS interviewers were only asked to carry out an initial, general investigation:

was there any possibility of the subject suffering from a psychotic illness? If further investigation was needed psychiatrists were asked to carry out a follow-up clinical interview. The questions for the initial investigation were pitched at such a level to reduce as far as possible the number of false negatives albeit at the cost of increasing the false positive rate.

Screening for psychosis included asking about presently occurring symptoms, but also asking informants directly what was the matter with them; whether they were taking anti-psychotic drugs or having anti-psychotic injections, and whether they had contact with any health care professional for a mental, nervous or emotional problem which had been labelled as a psychotic illness.

The sift for presently occurring symptoms, Psychosis Sift Questionnaire (PSQ), was developed specifically for this project.[4] The additional questions were added to minimise the false negative rate in the context of a disorder of low prevalence.

Clinicians who followed up potential cases were trained to carry out their interviews using SCAN (Schedules for Clinical Assessment in Neuropsychiatry) which is programmed on to a laptop computer.[5] SCAN is a set of instruments aimed at assessing, measuring and classifying the psychopathology and behaviour associated with the major psychiatric disorders of adult life. Of its four main components, the PSE10 was the one deemed most applicable for the purposes of this survey.[6] The PSE10 itself has two parts. Part One covers, inter alia, anxiety, depressive and bipolar disorders. Part Two includes the psychotic disorders of interest to the survey: schizophrenia, delusional and schizoaffective disorders, plus mania and affective bipolar disorder.

Because of the logistical difficulties in following up a mobile population throughout Great Britain with a psychiatric assessment, not everyone eligible for a SCAN interview was contacted. When a SCAN interview was done, those who were assessed as having psychosis in the past year were defined for this survey as a "definite" case of psychosis. If a SCAN interview was not done but the person screened positive in the OPCS interview because of self-reported psychosis or being prescribed antipsychotic medication, the OPCS survey data were reviewed. This involved collating coded responses and verbatim answers to create case studies. The topics included in this review were:

- age and sex of the subject
- subject's report of long-standing illness and onset of episode
- doctor's diagnosis of a mental, nervous or emotional problem as reported by the informant
- the subject's medication (including injections), dosage and compliance
- psychotic symptoms (as measured by the Psychosis Screening Questionnaire)
- CIS-R and GHQ12 scores (if available)
- Measures of alcohol and drug dependence (for residents of nightshelters and those using day centres)
- Use of mental health services (for residents of nightshelters and those using day centres)

Two psychiatric epidemiologists working independently were sent all the case studies for assessment. Based on this information they ascribed a diagnosis of psychosis with an indicator of certainty. If the subject was on antipsychotic medication, with an appropriate dosage, and the doctor was reported to have given a diagnosis of psychosis, this was regarded as giving a clear indication of psychosis. In other cases there was less certainty because the assessment was just based on one fact relating to their medication or what the subject said was the matter with them.

If subjects only screened positive for psychosis because of the response to the Psychosis Screening questionnaire, they were regarded as having a low likelihood of psychosis. This was based on evidence from the private household survey and borne out by results of SCAN interviews on the homeless survey.

For consistency, even those who were found not to have a psychotic illness after a SCAN interview were assessed as case studies. In a small number of these cases, the assessment of the case study indicated the presence of psychosis.

A summary of assessment procedures, the conditions for their applicability, and the range of consequences for each assessment is presented below. Only the three outcomes - definite, almost certain and fairly certain - are deemed to be cases of psychosis to be used in calculating prevalence rates.

Type of assessment	Applicability	Outcome
SCAN	Adults who screened positive for psychosis, with a SCAN positive result for psychosis	Definite
Case study	Adults who screened positive for psychosis (excluding those solely identified by the PSQ) who were SCAN negative for psychosis or did not have a SCAN interview	Almost certain or Fairly certain or Little certainty or Definitely not psychotic
No assessment	Adults who screened positive for psychosis solely identified by the PSQ	Very low likelihood assumed to be non-psychotic
	Adults who screened negative for psychosis	Definitely not psychotic

B5. Alcohol dependence

The twelve questions on alcohol dependence were taken from a national alcohol survey carried out in the USA in 1984. An anglicised version was created to measure the three components of dependence: loss of control, symptomatic behaviour and binge drinking.

Loss of control
Score one for positive response to each of:

1. Once I started drinking it was difficult for me to stop before I became completely drunk

2. I sometimes kept on drinking after I had promised myself not to.

3. I deliberately tried to cut down or stop drinking, but I was unable to do so.

4. Sometimes I have needed a drink so badly that I could not think of anything else.

Symptomatic behaviour
Score one for positive response to each of:

1. I have skipped a number of regular meals while drinking.

2. I have often had an alcoholic drink the first thing when I got up in the morning.

3. I have had a strong drink in the morning to get over the previous night's drinking.

4. I have woken up the next day not being able to remember some of the things I had done while drinking.

5. My hand shook a lot in the morning after drinking.

6. I need more alcohol than I used to get the same effect as before.

7. Sometimes I have woken up during the night or early morning sweating all over because of drinking.

Binge drinking
Score one for:

1. I have stayed drunk for several days at a time.

Although Room[1] originally had 13 items the same method of classifying severity of dependence was chosen:

0 items affirmed = no problem
1-2 items affirmed= minimal problem
3 or more items affirmed = at least a moderate problem
4 or more items affirmed = problem at a high level

For the tables in this report anyone with a score of 3 or more is deemed to have moderate alcohol dependence and those with a score of 7 or more have severe dependence.

B6. Drug dependence

A measure of drug dependence was derived from responses to a self-completion questionnaire asked of all survey respondents. Dependence was measured by regularity of drug use. Individuals were classified as drug dependent if they gave a positive response to the question: Have you ever used any one of these drugs every day for two weeks or more in the past 12 months?

The list of 10 categories of drug is shown in the box overleaf. A prerequisite was that the drugs must have been taken either without a prescription, more than what was prescribed for the subject, or to get high.

1. Sleeping Pills, Barbiturates, Sedatives, Downers, Seconal

2. Tranquillisers, Valium, Librium

3. Cannabis, Marijuana, Hash, Dope, Grass, Ganja, Kif

4. Amphetamines, Speed, Uppers, Stimulants, Qat

5. Cocaine, Coke, Crack

6. Heroin, Smack

7. Opiates other than heroin: Demerol, Morphine, Methadone, Darvon,Opium, DF118

8. Psychedelics, Hallucinogens: LSD, Mescaline, Acid, Peyote, Psylocybin (Magic) mushrooms

9. Ecstasy

10. Solvents, inhalants, glue, amyl nitrate

References

1. Clarke, W.B. and Hilton, M.E. (eds) (1991). *Alcohol in America: drinking practices and problems.* State University of New York Press, Albany.

Appendix C A comparison of the GHQ12 with the CIS-R

Because the revised Clinical Interview Schedule (CIS-R)[1] was not administered in nightshelters and day centres, all informants in each of the four homeless samples were asked to complete the GHQ12.[2] The purpose of this was that in hostels and PSLA, it would be possible to compare the GHQ12 with the CIS-R and determine the appropriate threshold score on the GHQ12 which corresponded with the case-defining threshold score used on the CIS-R.

In making comparisons between the instruments, it should be noted that the CIS-R measures the presence of neurotic disorder *during the past week* whereas the GHQ12 focuses on breaks in normal function such as the inability to continue to carry out one's normal 'healthy' functions, and the appearance of new phenomenon of a distressing nature *over the past few weeks.*

In hostels and PSLA, all 798 informants who had a personal interview answered both the GHQ12 and the CIS-R. There was no time delay in administering the two instruments, and in most cases the GHQ12 was completed before the CIS-R.

To compare the GHQ12 against the CIS-R, and to assess the effect of varying the threshold score we carried out receiver (or 'relative') operating characteristic (ROC) analysis. Two coefficients are plotted for all the possible

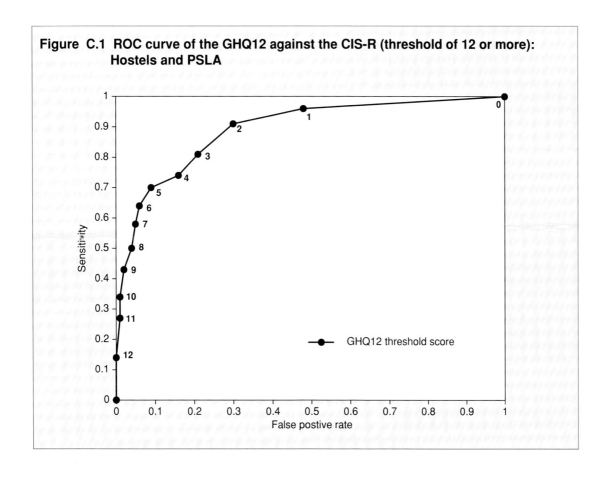

Figure C.1 ROC curve of the GHQ12 against the CIS-R (threshold of 12 or more): Hostels and PSLA

threshold levels of the GHQ12 using the definition of a case as having a CIS-R score of 12 or more:

a.   sensitivity - this is the proportion of CIS-R cases (defined as having a score of 12 or more) which are correctly identified by the GHQ12.

b.   false positive rate (or the complement of the specificity) - this is the proportion of cases identified by the GHQ12 which were not cases according to the CIS-R.

The ROC curve summarises the trade-off between sensitivity and the false positive rate as the threshold score on the GHQ is raised. Perfect agreement between the two instruments would be characterised by 100% sensitivity and 0% false positive rate.

In hostels and PSLA, 35% of adults were defined as cases by the CIS-R using a threshold score of 12 or more. By comparison, using a threshold score of 4 or more on the GHQ12, 37% of adults were defined as cases. At this threshold level, sensitivity was 74% and the false positive rate was 14%. That is, using a cut off of 4 or more on the GHQ12, the GHQ12 correctly identifies 74% of cases as defined by the CIS-R, but also misclassifies 14% of those who were not CIS-R cases.

Similarly, a threshold score of 6 or more on the GHQ12 was found to correspond with the higher CIS-R threshold of 18 or more; 27% of adults had a GHQ12 score of 6 or more and 26% of adults had a CIS-R score of 18 or more. At this threshold level the sensitivity was found to be 64% and the false positive rate was 10%.

Hence, two thresholds were determined for the GHQ12:

CIS-R threshold:	12	18
Corresponding GHQ12 threshold:	4	6

References

1   Lewis, G. and Pelosi, A.J., *Manual of the Revised Clinical Interview Schedule, (CIS-R)*, June 1990, Institute of Psychiatry. See also Lewis, G., Pelosi, A.J., Araya, R.C. and Dunn, G., (1992) Measuring psychiatric disorder in the community: a standardized assessment for use by lay interviewers, *Psychological Medicine*, **22**, 465-486.

2   Goldberg, D. and Williams, PA., (1988) *User's Guide to the General Health Questionnaire*, NFER-NELSON

Appendix D The survey documents

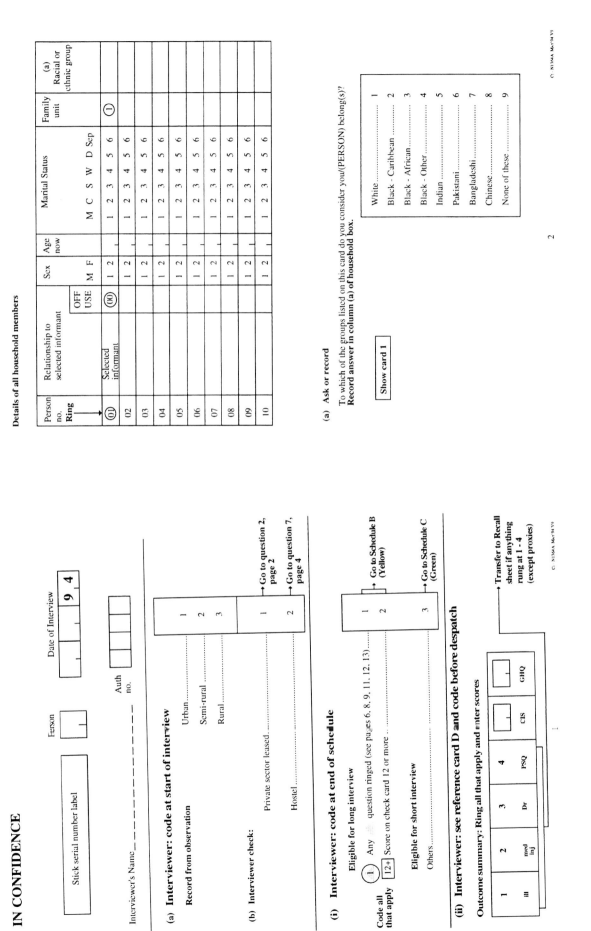

2 Private Sector Leased only

Details of all household members

Person no. Ring →	Relationship to selected informant		Sex M F	Age now	Marital Status M C S W D Sep	Family unit	(a) Racial or ethnic group
		OFF USE					
⑪	Selected informant	⑩	1 2	—	1 2 3 4 5 6	①	
02			1 2	—	1 2 3 4 5 6		
03			1 2	—	1 2 3 4 5 6		
04			1 2	—	1 2 3 4 5 6		
05			1 2	—	1 2 3 4 5 6		
06			1 2	—	1 2 3 4 5 6		
07			1 2	—	1 2 3 4 5 6		
08			1 2	—	1 2 3 4 5 6		
09			1 2	—	1 2 3 4 5 6		
10			1 2	—	1 2 3 4 5 6		

(a) Ask or record

To which of the groups listed on this card do you consider you/(PERSON) belong(s)?
Record answer in column (a) of household box.

Show card 1

White	1
Black - Caribbean	2
Black - African	3
Black - Other	4
Indian	5
Pakistani	6
Bangladeshi	7
Chinese	8
None of these	9

2

© N1364 Ma/94 V9

A

N1364   **Hostels and PSL Sift Schedule**

IN CONFIDENCE

	Person	Date of Interview
Stick serial number label		9 4

Interviewer's Name _ _ _ _ _ _ _ _   Auth no. _ _ _ _ _

1. (a) Interviewer: code at start of interview

Record from observation

Urban 1
Semi-rural 2
Rural 3

(b) Interviewer check:

Private sector leased .... 1 → **Go to Schedule B (Yellow)**
.... 2

Hostel .... 3 → **Go to Schedule C (Green)**

(i) Interviewer: code at end of schedule

Eligible for long interview

Code all that apply
① Any ▨ question ringed (see pages 6, 8, 9, 11, 12, 13) .... → **Go to question 2, page 2**
[12+] Score on check card 12 or more .... → **Go to question 7, page 4**

Eligible for short interview

Others ....

(ii) Interviewer: see reference card D and code before despatch

Outcome summary: Ring all that apply and enter scores

1	2	3	4
ill	med inj	Dr	PSQ

CIS	GHQ

→ **Transfer to Recall sheet if anything rung at 1 - 4 (except proxies)**

1

© N1364 Ma/94 V9

7   Hostels only

Details of selected person and family if living together

Person no. Ring →	Relationship to selected informant	Sex M F	Age now	Marital Status M C S W D Scp						Family unit	(a) Racial or ethnic group
				1	2	3	4	5	6		
(01)	Selected informant	(00) OFF USE 1 2	—	1	2	3	4	5	6	(1)	
02		1 2	—	1	2	3	4	5	6		
03		1 2	—	1	2	3	4	5	6		
04		1 2	—	1	2	3	4	5	6		
05		1 2	—	1	2	3	4	5	6		
06		1 2	—	1	2	3	4	5	6		
07		1 2	—	1	2	3	4	5	6		
08		1 2	—	1	2	3	4	5	6		
09		1 2	—	1	2	3	4	5	6		
10		1 2	—	1	2	3	4	5	6		

(a) **Ask or record**

To which of the groups listed on this card do you consider you/(PERSON) belong(s)?
Record answer in column (a) of family box.

Show card 1

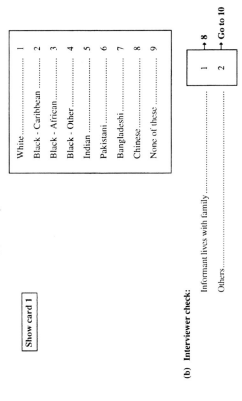

White 1
Black - Caribbean ... 2
Black - African 3
Black - Other 4
Indian 5
Pakistani 6
Bangladeshi 7
Chinese 8
None of these 9

(b) **Interviewer check:**

Informant lives with family .... 1 → 8
Others .... 2 → Go to 10

4

---

3   Household check :

Code from household box

Interviewer code: number of children (aged under 16) →
Interviewer code: number of adults aged 16 to 64 →
Interviewer code: number of adults aged 65 or more →

4 Now I would like to ask you a few questions about your accommodation.

Ask or record

How many bedrooms does your household have, including bedsitting rooms?

Include spare bedrooms available for informant's use
Exclude bedrooms converted to other uses

1 - 8 Enter No →
9 or more 9

5 How long have you been living in this flat/house?

Less than 3 months 1
3 months but less than 6 months 2
6 months but less than 1 year 3
1 year but less than 2 years 4
2 years but less than 3 years 5
3 years or more 6

6 Do you expect to move from here in the next 6 months?

Yes ..... 1 → (a)
No/Dk ... 2 → Go to 13, page 6

(a) (Can I check), why is that?

Code first that applies

Probe where necessary

Expecting permanent housing .... 1 → Go to 13, page 6
Expecting to move to other temporary housing 2
Expect to move but Dk if permanent/temporary 3
Other reason 4

3

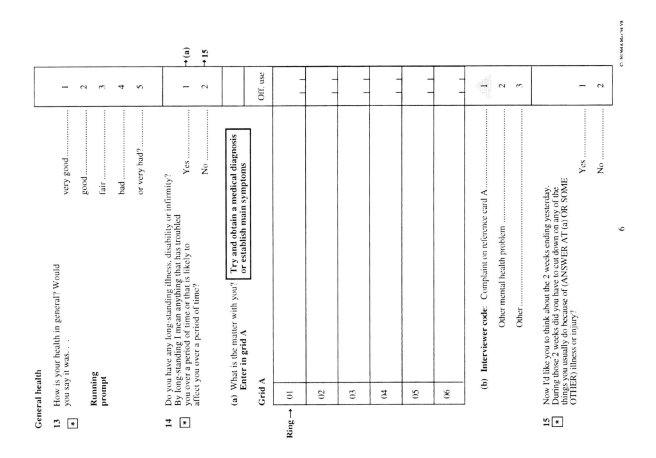

General health

13 How is your health in general? Would you say it was. . .

[*]

Running prompt

very good	1
good	2
fair	3
bad	4
or very bad?	5

14 Do you have any long-standing illness, disability or infirmity? By long-standing I mean anything that has troubled you over a period of time or that is likely to affect you over a period of time?

[*]

Yes	1	→ (a)
No	2	→ 15

(a) What is the matter with you? Enter in grid A

[Try and obtain a medical diagnosis or establish main symptoms]

Grid A

Ring →		Off. use
01		
02		
03		
04		
05		
06		

(b) **Interviewer code:**

Complaint on reference card A	1
Other mental health problem	2
Other	3

15 Now I'd like you to think about the 2 weeks ending yesterday. During those 2 weeks did you have to cut down on any of the things you usually do because of (ANSWER AT (a) OR SOME OTHER) illness or injury?

[*]

Yes	1
No	2

6

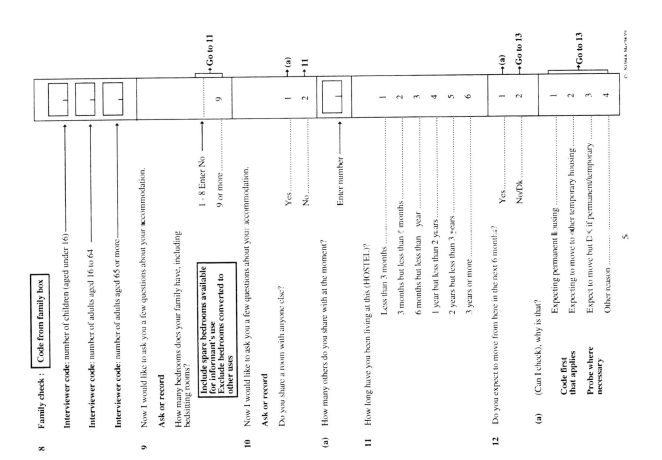

8 **Family check :** | Code from family box |

Interviewer code: number of children (aged under 16)

Interviewer code: number of adults aged 16 to 64

Interviewer code: number of adults aged 65 or more

9 Now I would like to ask you a few questions about your accommodation.

Ask or record

How many bedrooms does your family have, including bedsitting rooms?

Include spare bedrooms available for informant's use
Exclude bedrooms converted to other uses

1 - 8 Enter No	→ Go to 11
9 or more	9

10 Now I would like to ask you a few questions about your accommodation.

Ask or record

Do you share a room with anyone else?

Yes	1	→ (a)
No	2	→ 11

(a) How many others do you share with at the moment?

Enter number

11 How long have you been living at this (HOSTEL)?

Less than 3 months	1
3 months but less than 6 months	2
6 months but less than year	3
1 year but less than 2 years	4
2 years but less than 3 years	5
3 years or more	6

12 Do you expect to move from here in the next 6 months?

Yes	1	→ (a)
No/Dk	2	→ Go to 13

(a) (Can I check), why is that?

Code first that applies

Probe where necessary

Expecting permanent housing	1	→ Go to 13
Expecting to move to other temporary housing	2	
Expect to move but DK if permanent/temporary	3	→ Go to 13
Other reason	4	

5

157

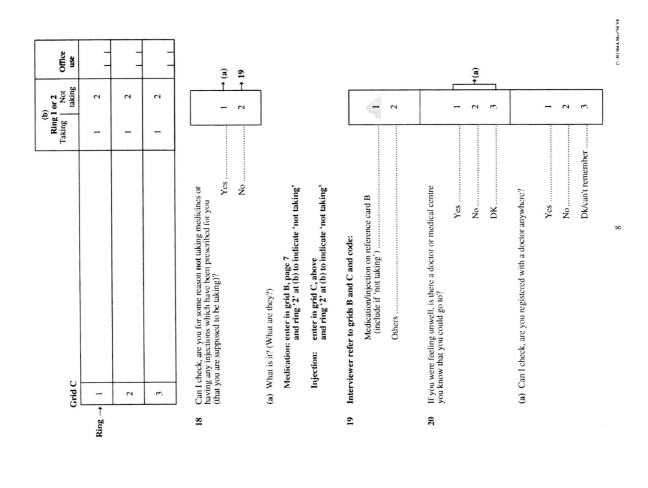

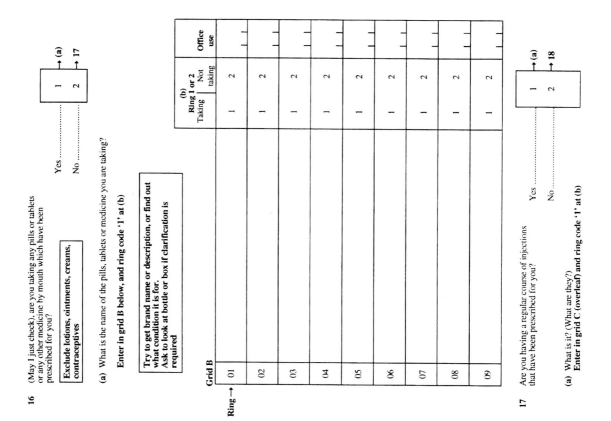

24 [*] Have you noticed a marked loss in your appetite in the past month?

Yes .... 1 → (a)
No .... 2 → 26

25 Have you lost any weight in the past month?

Yes .... 1 → 28
No/DK .... 2 → (b)

(a) Were you trying to lose weight or on a diet?

Yes .... 1 → 28
No 2

(b) Did you lose half a stone or more, or did you lose less than this?

| Half a stone or 7 lbs or 3¼ kg |

lost half a stone or more 1
lost less than half a stone .... 2 → 28

26 [*] Have you noticed a marked increase in your appetite in the past month?

Yes 1
No 2

27 Have you gained weight in the past month?

| Do not include weight gain due to pregnancy |

Yes 1
No/DK 2

28 Interviewer check: Interview with:

subject .... 1 → **Go to GH self completion then go to P1, page 11**
proxy .... 2 → **Complete front page**
both .... 3 → **Go to GH self completion for completion by subject; then go to P1, page 11**

10

G-N136A Me/94 V8

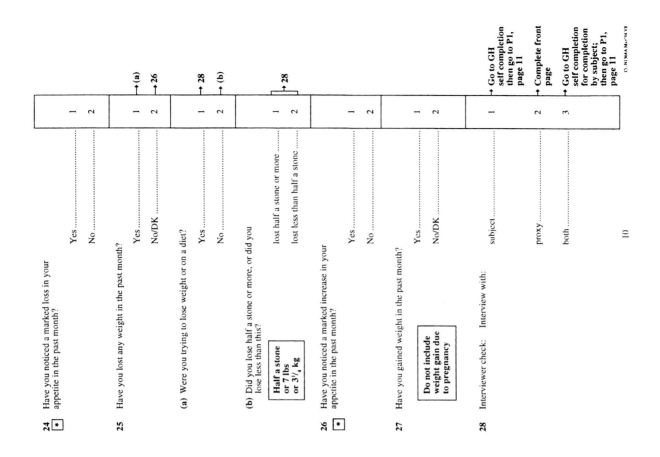

21 During the 2 weeks ending yesterday, apart from any visit to a hospital, did you talk to a doctor for any reason at all, either in person or by telephone?

Exclude: consultations made on behalf of children under 16 and persons not living with informant as family

Yes .... 1 → (a)
No .... 2 → 22

(a) How many times did you talk to a doctor in these 2 weeks?

Enter number → [ ]

22 In the past twelve months, have you spoken to a doctor on your own behalf, either in person or by telephone about a physical illness or complaint?

Yes 1
No 2

23 In the past twelve months have you spoken to a doctor on your own behalf, either in person or by telephone about being anxious or depressed or a mental, nervous or emotional problem?

Yes .... 1 → (a)
No .... 2 → 24

(a) What did the doctor say was the matter with you? **Enter in grid D**

Try and obtain a medical diagnosis or establish main symptoms

Grid D	Off. use
Ring → 01	
02	
03	
04	
05	
06	

(b) Interviewer code: Complaint on reference card A .... 1 → 24
Other mental health problem 2
Other 3

9

G-N136A Me/94 V8

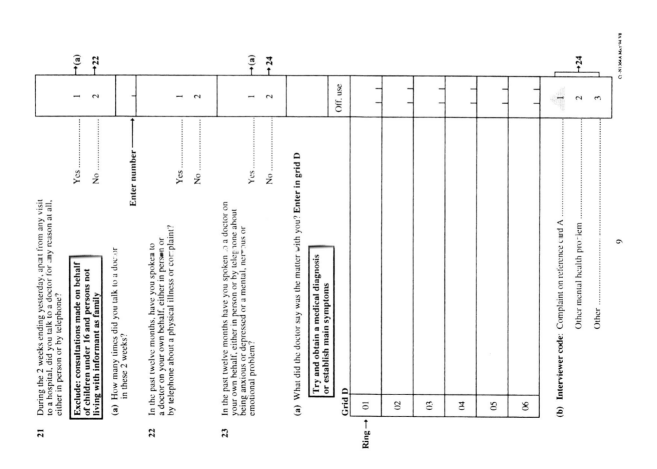

P.   **PSQ**

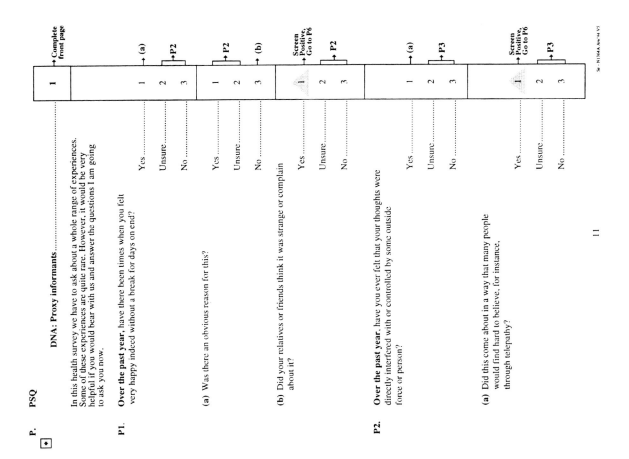

* DNA: Proxy informants .... | 1 | → Complete front page

In this health survey we have to ask about a whole range of experiences. Some of these experiences are quite rare. However, it would be very helpful if you would bear with us and answer the questions I am going to ask you now.

P1.   **Over the past year**, have there been times when you felt very happy indeed without a break for days on end?
Yes ...... 1 → (a)
Unsure ...... 2 → P2
No ...... 3 → P2

(a) Was there an obvious reason for this?
Yes ...... 1 → P2
Unsure ...... 2 → P2
No ...... 3 → (b)

(b) Did your relatives or friends think it was strange or complain about it?
Yes ...... 1 → Screen Positive, Go to P6
Unsure ...... 2 → P2
No ...... 3 → P2

P2.   **Over the past year**, have you ever felt that your thoughts were directly interfered with or controlled by some outside force or person?
Yes ...... 1 → (a)
Unsure ...... 2 → P3
No ...... 3 → P3

(a) Did this come about in a way that many people would find hard to believe, for instance, through telepathy?
Yes ...... 1 → Screen Positive, Go to P6
Unsure ...... 2 → P3
No ...... 3 → P3

Se - N1364A Apr'94 V5

11

P3.   **Over the past year**, have there been times when you felt that people were against you?
Yes ...... 1 → (a)
Unsure ...... 2 → P4
No 3

(a) Have there been times when you felt that people were deliberately acting to harm you or your interests?
Yes ...... 1 → (b)
Unsure ...... 2 → P4
No 3

(b) Have there been times you felt that a group of people was plotting to cause you serious harm or injury?
Yes ...... 1 → Screen Positive, Go to P6
Unsure ...... 2 → P4
No 3

P4   **Over the past year**, have there been times when you felt that something <u>strange</u> was going on?
Yes ...... 1 → (a)
Unsure ...... 2 → P5
No 3

(a) Did you feel it was so strange that other people would find it very hard to believe?
Yes ...... 1 → Screen Positive, Go to P6
Unsure ...... 2 → P5
No 3

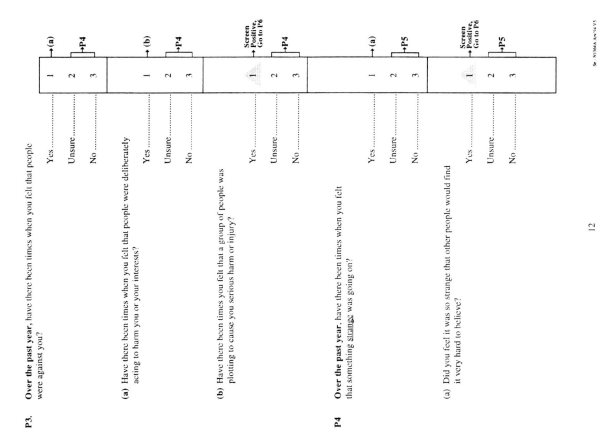

Se - N1364A Apr'94 V5

12

P5. **Over the past year**, have there been times when you heard or saw things that other people couldn't?

Yes .... 1 → (a)
Unsure .... 2 → Screen Negative, Go to P6
No .... 3 → Screen Negative, Go to P6

a) Did you at any time hear voices saying quite a few words or sentences when there was no one around that might account for it?

Yes .... 1 → Screen Positive, Go to P6
Unsure .... 2 → Screen Negative Go to P6
No .... 3 → Screen Negative Go to P6

P6. **Interviewer check**

Informant screened positive .... 1 → Go to Section A (CIS-R) page 14
Informant screened negative 2

13

CIS - R

[*] A Somatic symptoms

A1 Have you had any sort of ache or pain in the past month?

Yes .... 1 → A3
No .... 2 → A2

A2 During the past month have you been troubled by any sort of discomfort, for example, headache or indigestion?

Yes .... 1 → A3
No .... 2 → Go to section B

A3 Was this ache or pain/discomfort brought on or made worse because you were feeling low, anxious or stressed?

Yes .... 1 → A4
No .... 2 → Go to Section B

> **If informant has more than one pain/discomfort, refer to ANY of them**

A4 In the past seven days, including last (DAY OF WEEK), on how many days have you noticed the ache or pain/discomfort?

4 days or more .... 1 → A5
1 to 3 days 2
None .... 3 → A9

A5 In total, did the ache or pain/discomfort last for more than 3 hours on any day in the past week/on that day?

Yes 1
No 2

14

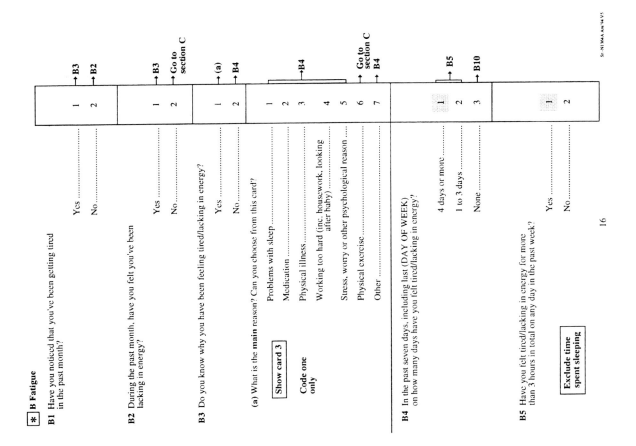

* B Fatigue

B1 Have you noticed that you've been getting tired in the past month?

Yes ... 1 → **B3**
No ... 2 → **B2**

B2 During the past month, have you felt you've been lacking in energy?

Yes ... 1 → **B3**
No ... 2 → **Go to section C**

B3 Do you know why you have been feeling tired/lacking in energy?

Yes ... 1 → **(a)**
No ... 2 → **B4**

(a) What is the **main** reason? Can you choose from this card?

Show card 3

Code one only

Problems with sleep ... 1 → **B4**
Medication ... 2
Physical illness ... 3
Working too hard (inc. housework, looking after baby) ... 4
Stress, worry or other psychological reason ... 5 → **Go to section C**
Physical exercise ... 6 → **B4**
Other ... 7

B4 In the past seven days, including last (DAY OF WEEK) on how many days have you felt tired/lacking in energy?

4 days or more ... 1 → **B5**
1 to 3 days ... 2
None ... 3 → **B10**

B5 Have you felt tired/lacking in energy for more than 3 hours in total on any day in the past week?

Yes ... 1
No ... 2

Exclude time spent sleeping

Sr. N1366A Aw '94 V5

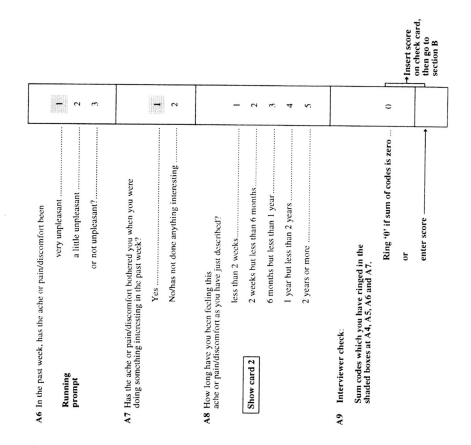

A6 In the past week, has the ache or pain/discomfort been

Running prompt

very unpleasant ... 1
a little unpleasant ... 2
or not unpleasant? ... 3

A7 Has the ache or pain/discomfort bothered you when you were doing something interesting in the past week?

Yes ... 1
No/has not done anything interesting ... 2

A8 How long have you been feeling this ache or pain/discomfort as you have just described?

Show card 2

less than 2 weeks ... 1
2 weeks but less than 6 months ... 2
6 months but less than 1 year ... 3
1 year but less than 2 years ... 4
2 years or more ... 5

A9 Interviewer check:

Sum codes which you have ringed in the shaded boxes at A4, A5, A6 and A7.

Ring '0' if sum of codes is zero ... 0

or

enter score → **Insert score on check card, then go to section B**

Sr. N1366A Aw '94 V5

✱ C Concentration and forgetfulness

C1 In the past month, have you had any problems in concentrating on what you are doing?

Yes, problems concentrating	1
No	2

C2 Have you noticed any problems with forgetting things in the past month?

Yes	1
No	2

C3 Interviewer code

Informant has problems concentrating or forgets things (coded 1 at C1 or C2)	1	→ **C4**
Others	2	→ **Go to section D**

C4 Since last (DAY OF WEEK), on how many days have you noticed problems with your concentration/memory?

4 days or more	1	→ **C5**
1 to 3 days	2	
None	3	→ **C9**

C5 Informants who had concentration problems

DNA: others (coded 2 at C1)	1	→ **C7**

In the past week could you concentrate on a TV programme, read a newspaper article or talk to someone without your mind wandering?

Yes	2
No/not always	1

C6 In the past week, have these problems with your concentration actually **stopped** you from getting on with things you used to do or would like to do?

Yes	1
No	2

18

B6 Have you felt so tired/lacking in energy that you've had to push yourself to get things done during the past week?

Yes, on at least one occasion	1
No	2 → **B9**

B7 Have you felt tired/lacking in energy when doing things that you enjoy during the past week?

Yes, at least once	1
No	2
Spontaneous Does not enjoy anything	3 → **B8**

B8 Have you in the past week felt tired/lacking in energy when doing things that you **used** to enjoy?

Yes	1
No	2

B9 How long have you been feeling tired/lacking in energy in the way you have just described?

Show card 2

less than 2 weeks	1
2 weeks but less than 6 months	2
6 months but less than 1 year	3
1 year but less than 2 years	4
2 years or more	5

B10 Interviewer check:

Sum codes which you have ringed in the shaded boxes at B4, B5, B6, B7 and B8.

Ring '0' if sum of codes is zero	0

→ **Insert score on check card, then go to section C**

or

enter score ⟶

17

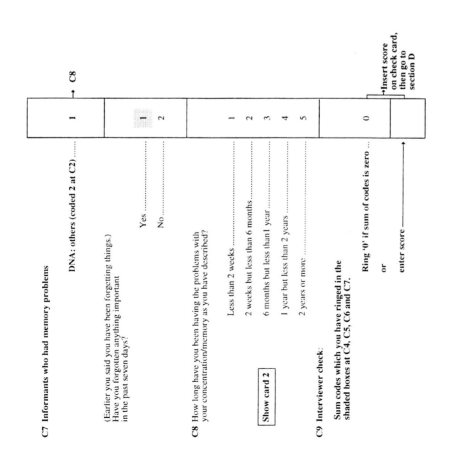

C7 Informants who had memory problems

DNA: others (coded 2 at C2) .... 1 → C8

(Earlier you said you have been forgetting things.) Have you forgotten anything important in the past seven days?

Yes 1
No 2

C8 How long have you been having the problems with your concentration/memory as you have described?

| Show card 2 |

Less than 2 weeks 1
2 weeks but less than 6 months 2
6 months but less than 1 year 3
1 year but less than 2 years 4
2 years or more 5

C9 Interviewer check:

Sum codes which you have ringed in the shaded boxes at C4, C5, C6 and C7.

Ring '0' if sum of codes is zero 0

or

enter score ———— → **Insert score on check card, then go to section D**

19

---

* D Sleep problems

D1 In the past month, have you been having problems with trying to get to sleep or with getting back to sleep if you woke up or were woken up?

Yes .... 1 → D3
No .... 2 → D2

D2 Has sleeping more than you usually do been a problem for you in the past month?

Yes .... 1 → D3
No .... 2 → Go to section E

D3 On how many of the past seven nights did you have problems with your sleep?

4 nights or more .... 1 → D4
1 to 3 nights 2
None .... 3 → D11

D4 Do you know why you are having problems with your sleep?

Yes .... 1 → (a)
No .... 2 → D5

(a) Can you look at this card and tell me the **main** reason for these problems?

| Show card 4 |

Code one only

Noise 1
Shift work/too busy to sleep 2
Illness/discomfort 3
Worry/thinking 4
Needing to go to the toilet 5
Having to do something (e.g. look after baby) . 6
Tired 7
Medication 8
Other 9

20

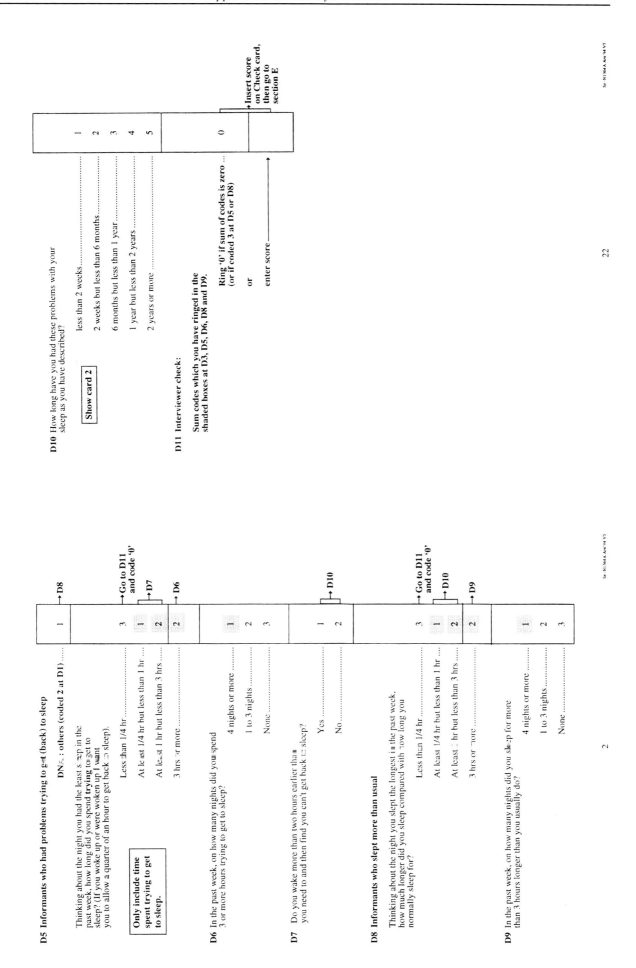

D5 Informants who had problems trying to get (back) to sleep

DNA: others (coded 2 at D1) .... 1 → D8

Thinking about the night you had the least sleep in the past week, how long did you spend **trying** to get to sleep? (**If you woke up or were woken up I want you to allow a quarter of an hour to get back to sleep**).

| Only include time spent trying to get to sleep. |

Less than 1/4 hr .... 3 → Go to D11 and code '0'

At least 1/4 hr but less than 1 hr .... 1 → D7

At least 1 hr but less than 3 hrs 2

3 hrs or more .... 2 → D6

D6 In the past week, on how many nights did you spend 3 or more hours trying to get to sleep?

4 nights or more 1

1 to 3 nights 2

None 3

D7 Do you wake more than two hours earlier than you need to and then find you can't get back to sleep?

Yes .... 1 → D10

No 2

D8 Informants who slept more than usual

Thinking about the night you slept the longest in the past week, how much longer did you sleep compared with how long you normally sleep for?

Less than 1/4 hr .... 3 → Go to D11 and code '0'

At least 1/4 hr but less than 1 hr .... 1 → D10

At least 1 hr but less than 3 hrs 2

3 hrs or more .... 2 → D9

D9 In the past week, on how many nights did you sleep for more than 3 hours longer than you usually do?

4 nights or more 1

1 to 3 nights 2

None 3

D10 How long have you had these problems with your sleep as you have described?

| Show card 2 |

less than 2 weeks 1

2 weeks but less than 6 months 2

6 months but less than 1 year 3

1 year but less than 2 years 4

2 years or more 5

D11 Interviewer check:

Sum codes which you have ringed in the shaded boxes at D3, D5, D6, D8 and D9.

Ring '0' if sum of codes is zero (or if coded 3 at D5 or D8) 0

or

enter score →

→ **Insert score on Check card, then go to section E**

22

2

Sr: N1364A Am'94 V5

165

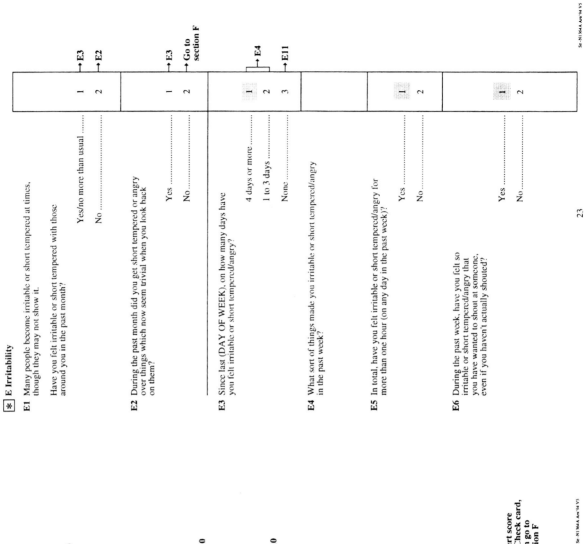

✱ E Irritability

E1 Many people become irritable or short tempered at times, though they may not show it.

Have you felt irritable or short tempered with those around you in the past month?

Yes/no more than usual	1 → E3
No	2 → E2

E2 During the past month did you get short tempered or angry over things which now seem trivial when you look back on them?

Yes	1 → E3
No	2 → Go to section F

E3 Since last (DAY OF WEEK), on how many days have you felt irritable or short tempered/angry?

4 days or more	1 ⎤
1 to 3 days	2 ⎦ → E4
None	3 → E11

E4 What sort of things made you irritable or short tempered/angry in the past week?

E5 In total, have you felt irritable or short tempered/angry for more than one hour (on any day in the past week)?

Yes	1
No	2

E6 During the past week, have you felt so irritable or short tempered/angry that you have wanted to shout at someone, even if you haven't actually shouted?

Yes	1
No	2

23

Sr-N1364A Apr'94 V5

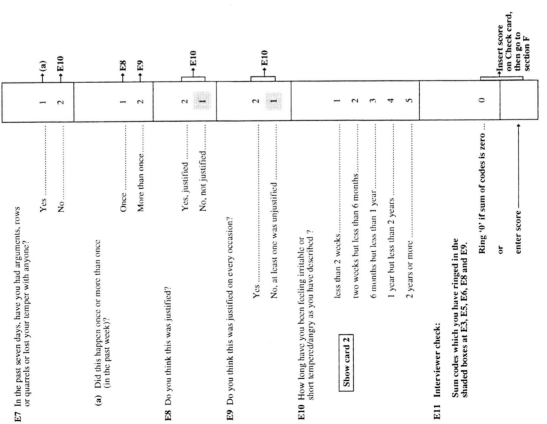

E7 In the past seven days, have you had arguments, rows or quarrels or lost your temper with anyone?

Yes	1 → (a)
No	2 → E10

(a) Did this happen once or more than once (in the past week)?

Once	1 → E8
More than once	2 → E9

E8 Do you think this was justified?

Yes, justified	2
No, not justified	1 → E10

E9 Do you think this was justified on every occasion?

Yes	2
No, at least one was unjustified	1 → E10

E10 How long have you been feeling irritable or short tempered/angry as you have described ?

Show card 2

less than 2 weeks	1
two weeks but less than 6 months	2
6 months but less than 1 year	3
1 year but less than 2 years	4
2 years or more	5

E11 Interviewer check:

Sum codes which you have ringed in the shaded boxes at E3, E5, E6, E8 and E9.

Ring '0' if sum of codes is zero ... 0 → Insert score on Check card, then go to section F

or

enter score →

24

Sr-N1364A Apr'94 V5

166

[*] F Worry about physical health

F1 Many people get concerned about their physical health. In the past month, have you been at all worried about your physical health?

Yes, worried	1	→ F3
No/concerned	2	→ F2

> Include women who are worried about their pregnancy

F2 Informants who have no problems with physical health

> DNA : has a physical health problem shown at 14a, page 6

	1	→ Go to section G

During the past month, did you find yourself worrying that you might have a serious physical illness?

Yes	1	→ F3
No	2	→ Go to section G

F3 Thinking about the past seven days, including last (DAY OF WEEK), on how many days have you found yourself worrying about your physical health/that you might have a serious physical illness?

4 days or more	1	→ F4
1 to 3 days	2	
None	3	→ F8

F4 In your opinion, have you been worrying too much in view of your actual health?

Yes	1
No	2

F5 In the past week, has this worrying been

Running prompt

very unpleasant	1
a little unpleasant	2
or not unpleasant?	3

F6 In the past week, have you been able to take your mind off your health worries at least once, by doing something else?

Yes	2
No, could not be distracted once	1

F7 How long have you been worrying about your physical health in the way you have described?

> Show card 2

less than 2 weeks	1
2 weeks but less than 6 months	2
6 months but less than 1 year	3
1 year but less than 2 years	4
2 years or more	5

F8 Interviewer check:

Sum codes which you have ringed in the shaded boxes at F3, F4, F5 and F6.

Ring '0' if sum of codes is zero	0
or	
enter score →	

→ Insert score on Check card, then go to section G

Se:NI364A Apr'94 V5

G Depression

G1 Almost everyone becomes sad, miserable or depressed at times.
Have you had a spell of feeling sad, miserable or depressed in the past month?

Yes 1
No 2

G2 During the past month, have you been able to enjoy or take an interest in things as much as you usually do?

Yes 1
No/no enjoyment or interest 2

G3 Interviewer check:

Code first that applies

Informant felt sad, miserable or depressed (coded 1 at G1) .... 1 → **G4**
Informant unable to enjoy or take an interest (coded 2 at G2) .... 2 → **G5**
Others .... 3 → **Go to Section I, page 32**

G4 In the past week have you had a spell of feeling sad, miserable or depressed?

Use informant's own words if possible

Yes 1
No .... 2 → **See G5**

G5 Informants who were unable to enjoy or take an interest in things

DNA: coded 1 at G2 .... 1 → **See G6**

In the past week have you been able to enjoy or take an interest in things as much as usual?

Use informant's own words if possible

Yes 2
No/no enjoyment or interest 1

G6 **Informants who felt sad, miserable or depressed or unable to enjoy or take an interest in things in the past week (coded 1 at G4 or G5)**

DNA: others .... 1 → **Go to G11**

Since last (DAY OF WEEK) on how many days have you felt sad, miserable or depressed/unable to enjoy or take an interest in things?

4 days or more 1
2 to 3 days 2
1 day 3

G7 Have you felt sad, miserable or depressed/unable to enjoy or take an interest in things for more than 3 hours in total (on any day in the past week)?

Yes 1
No 2

G8 (a) What sorts of things made you feel sad, miserable or depressed/unable to enjoy or take an interest in things in the past week? Can you choose from this card?

Ring code(s) in column (a).

Show card 5

	(a) Code all that apply	(b) Code one only
Members of the family	01	01
Relationship with spouse/partner	02	02
Relationships with friends	03	03
Housing	04	04
Money/bills	05	05
Own physical health (inc. pregnancy)	06	06
Own mental health	07	07
Work or lack of work (inc. student)	08	08
Legal difficulties	09	09
Political issues/the news	10	10
Other	11	11
Don't know/no main thing	99	99

(b) **DNA : Only one item coded at (a)** .... 1 → **G9**

What was the main thing?
Ring code in column (b)

Right section

* H Depressive Ideas

H1 Informants who scored 1 or more at section G, Depression

DNA: Others (coded 0 or blank at G11) ...... 1 → **Go to section I**

I would now like to ask you about when you have been feeling sad, miserable or depressed/unable to enjoy or take an interest in things. In the past week, was this worse in the morning or in the evening, or did this make no difference?

Prompt as necessary
in the morning 1
in the evening 2
no difference/other 3

H2 | Ask or use card 7 |

Many people find that feeling sad, miserable or depressed/unable to enjoy or take an interest in things can affect their interest in sex. Over the past month, do you think your interest in sex has

Running prompt
increased 1
decreased 2
or has it stayed the same? 3
Spontaneous Not applicable 4

	Yes	No
H3 When you have felt sad, miserable or depressed/unable to enjoy or take an interest in things in the past seven days, have you been so restless that you couldn't sit still?	1	2
Individual prompt have you been doing things more slowly, for example, walking more slowly?	1	2
have you been less talkative than normal?	1	2

H4 Now, thinking about the past seven days have you on at least one occasion felt guilty or blamed yourself when things went wrong when it **hasn't** been your fault?
Yes, at least once 1
No 2

H5 During the past week, have you been feeling you are not as good as other people?
Yes 1
No 2

H6 Have you felt hopeless at all during the past seven days, for instance about your future?
Yes 1
No 2

30

Left section

G9 In the past week when you felt sad, miserable or depressed/unable to enjoy or take an interest in things, did you ever become happier when something nice happened, or when you were in company?
Yes, at least once 2
No 1

G10 How long have you been feeling sad, miserable or depressed/unable to enjoy or take an interest in things as you have described?

| Show card 6 |
less than 2 weeks 1
2 weeks but less than 6 months 2
6 months but less than 1 year 3
1 year but less than 2 years 4
2 years or more 5

G11 Interviewer check:
Sum codes which you have ringed in the shaded boxes at G5, G6, G7 and G9.
Ring '0' if sum of codes is zero 0
or
enter score →

→ **Insert score on Check card, then go to section H**

29

(Page 32 — I Worry)

* I Worry

I 1 (The next few questions are about worrying.) In the past month, did you find yourself worrying more than you needed to about things?

Yes, worrying	1	→ I3
No/concerned	2	→ I2

I 2 Have you had any worries at all in the past month?

Yes	1	→ I3
No	2	→ Go to section J

I 3 (a) Can you look at this card and tell me what sorts of things you worried about in the past month?

Ring code(s) in column (a).

Show card 10

	(a) Code all that apply	(b) Code one only
Members of the family	01	01
Relationship with spouse/partner	02	02
Relationships with friends	03	03
Housing	04	04
Money/bills	05	05
Own physical health (inc. pregnancy)	06	06
Own mental health	07	07
Work or lack of work (inc student)	08	08
Legal difficulties	09	09
Political issues/the news	10	10
Other	11	11
Don't know/no main thing	99	99

(b) DNA : Only one item coded at (a) .... 1 → I4

What was the main thing you worried about?
Ring code in column (b).

I 4 Interviewer check:

Informant worries about physical health (coded 06 at I3(a))	1	See instruction below, then go to I5
Others (not coded 06 at I3(a))	2	→ I6

Make a note on Check flap to go to section F to record this worry about physical health, if not already recorded.

(Page 31)

H7 Interviewer check

Informant felt guilty, not as good as others or hopeless (coded 1 at H4 or H5 or H6)	1	→ H8
Others (coded 2 at H4, H5 and H6)	2	→ read H10

H8 [Ask or use card 8]

In the past week have you felt that life isn't worth living?

Yes	1	→ H9
Spontaneous: Yes, but not in the past week	2	→ read H10
No	3	

H9 [Ask or use card 9]

In the past week, have you thought of killing yourself?

Yes	1	→ (a)
Spontaneous: Yes, but not in the past week	2	→ read H10
No	3	

(a) Have you talked to your doctor about these thoughts (of killing yourself)?

Yes	1	→ read H10
Spontaneous: No, but has talked to other people	2	→ read (b)
No	3	

(b) (You have said that you are thinking about committing suicide.)

Since this is a very serious matter it is important that you talk to your doctor about these thoughts. → read H10

H10 (Thank you for answering those questions on how you have been feeling. I would now like to ask you a few questions about worrying.)

H11 Interviewer check:

Sum codes which you have ringed in the shaded boxes at H4, H5, H6, H8 and H9.

Ring '0' if sum of codes is zero	0	Insert score on Check card, then go to section I
or		
enter score _____		

Maximum score on this section is 5

I 10 How long have you been worrying about things in the way that you have described?

Show card 11

less than 2 weeks	1
2 weeks but less than 6 months	2
6 months but less than 1 year	3
1 year but less than 2 years	4
2 years or more	5

I 11 Interviewer check:
Sum codes which you have ringed in the shaded boxes at 16, 17, 18 and 19.

Ring '0' if sum of codes is zero ... 0

or

enter score ——→

→ **Insert score on Check card, then go to section J**

I 5 Interviewer check:

Informant is **only** worried about physical health (only code 06 is rung at I3 (a)) .... 1 → **Go to section J**

Informant had other worries (I3(a) is multi-coded) .... 2 → **read (a)**

(a) For the next few questions, I want you to think about the worries you have had **other** than those about your physical health.

I 6 On how many of the past seven days have you been worrying about things (other than your physical health)?

4 days or more .... 1 → **I7**
1 to 3 days 2
None .... 3 → **I11**

I 7 In your opinion, have you been worrying too much in view of your circumstances?

Yes 1
No 2

[Refer to worries other than those about physical health]

I 8 In the past week, has this worrying been:

Running prompt

very unpleasant 1
a little unpleasant 2
or not unpleasant? 3

[Refer to worries other than those about physical health]

I 9 Have you worried for more than 3 hours in total on any one of the past seven days?

Yes 1
No 2

[Refer to worries other than those about physical health]

★ J Anxiety

J1 Have you been feeling anxious or nervous in the past month?

Yes, anxious or nervous	1 → J3
No	2 → J2

J2 In the past month, did you ever find your muscles felt tense or that you couldn't relax?

Yes	1
No	2

J3 Some people have phobias; they get nervous or uncomfortable about specific things or situations when there is no real danger. For instance they may get nervous when speaking or eating in front of strangers, when they are far from home or in crowded rooms, or they may have a fear of heights. Others become nervous at the sight of things like blood or spiders.

In the past month have you felt anxious, nervous or tense about any specific things or situations when there was no real danger?

Yes	1
No	2

J4 Interviewer check:

Informant reports anxiety and also a phobia (coded 1 at J1 or J2, and coded 1 at J3)	1 → J5
Informant reports only general anxiety (coded 1 at J1 or J2, and coded 2 at J3)	2 → J7
Others	3 → Go to section K

J5 In the past month, when you felt anxious/nervous/tense, was this always brought on by the phobia about some specific situation or thing or did you sometimes feel generally anxious/nervous/tense?

Always brought on by phobia	1 → Go to section K
Sometimes felt generally anxious	2 → J6

J6 The next questions are concerned with **general anxiety/nervousness/tension only.** I will ask you about the anxiety which is brought on by the phobia about specific things or situations later.

On how many of the past seven days have you felt **generally** anxious/nervous/tense?

4 days or more	1 ⎫ → J8
1 to 3 days	2 ⎭
None	3 → J12

J7 On how many of the past seven days have you felt generally anxious/nervous/tense?

4 days or more	1 ⎫ → J8
1 to 3 days	2 ⎭
None	3 → J12

J8 In the past week, has your anxiety/nervousness/tension been:

Running prompt

very unpleasant	1
a little unpleasant	2
or not unpleasant?	3

J9 In the past week, when you've been anxious/nervous/tense, have you had any of the symptoms shown on this card?

Show card 12

Yes	1 → (a)
No	2 → J10

(a) Which of these symptoms did you have when you felt anxious/nervous/tense?

Code all that apply

Heart racing or pounding	1
Hands sweating or shaking	2
Feeling dizzy	3
Difficulty getting your breath	4
Butterflies in stomach	5
Dry mouth	6
Nausea or feeling as though you wanted to vomit	7

If informant had any of these symptoms, check J9 is coded 1, 'Yes'.

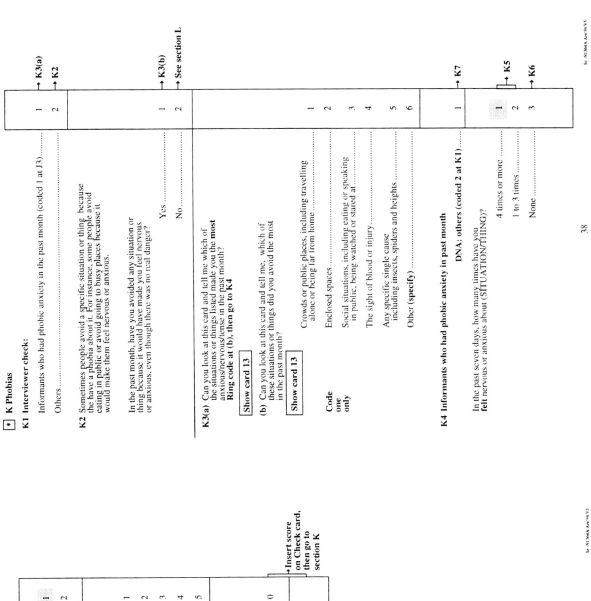

J10 Have you felt anxious/nervous/tense for more than 3 hours in total on any one of the past seven days?

Yes 1

No 2

J11 How long have you had these feelings of general anxiety/nervousness/tension as you described?

Show card 11

less than 2 weeks 1

2 weeks but less than 6 months 2

6 months but less than 1 year 3

1 year but less than 2 years 4

2 years or more 5

J12 Interviewer check:

Sum codes which you have ringed in the shaded boxes at J6, J7, J8, J9 and J10.

Ring '0' if sum of codes is zero ... 0

or

enter score _____

→**Insert score on Check card, then go to section K**

37

Se-NL364A Am'94 V5

⬜* **K Phobias**

K1 Interviewer check:

Informants who had phobic anxiety in the past month (coded 1 at J3) .... 1 → K3(a)

Others .... 2 → K2

K2 Sometimes people avoid a specific situation or thing because they have a phobia about it. For instance, some people avoid eating in public or avoid going to busy places because it would make them feel nervous or anxious.

In the past month, have you avoided any situation or thing because it would have made you feel nervous or anxious, even though there was no real danger?

Yes .... 1 → K3(b)

No .... 2 → See section L

K3(a) Can you look at this card and tell me which of the situations or things listed made you the **most** anxious/nervous/tense in the past month? **Ring code at (b), then go to K4**

Show card 13

(b) Can you look at this card and tell me, which of these situations or things did you avoid the most in the past month?

Show card 13

Code
one
only

Crowds or public places, including travelling alone or being far from home 1

Enclosed spaces 2

Social situations, including eating or speaking in public, being watched or stared at 3

The sight of blood or injury 4

Any specific single cause including insects, spiders and heights 5

Other (specify) 6

K4 Informants who had phobic anxiety in past month

DNA: others (coded 2 at K1) .... 1 → K7

In the past seven days, how many times have you felt nervous or anxious about (SITUATION/THING)?

4 times or more .... 1 → K5

1 to 3 times 2

None .... 3 → K6

38

Se-NL364A Am'94 V5

173

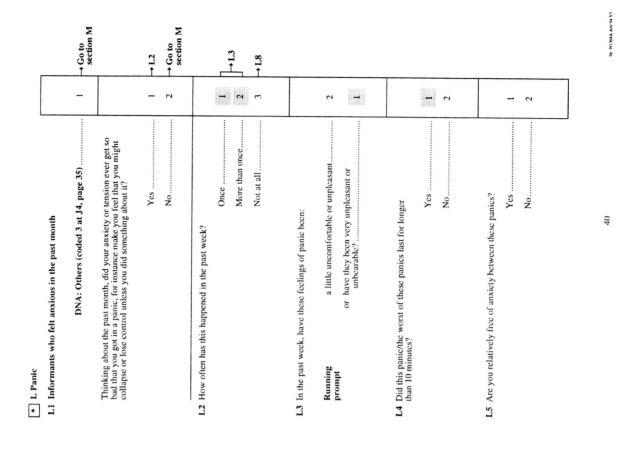

* L Panic

L1 Informants who felt anxious in the past month

DNA: Others (coded 3 at J4, page 35) .... 1 → Go to section M

Thinking about the past month, did your anxiety or tension ever get so bad that you got in a panic, for instance make you feel that you might collapse or lose control unless you did something about it?

Yes .... 1 → L2
No .... 2 → Go to section M

L2 How often has this happened in the past week?

Once .... 1 ⎤
More than once .... 2 ⎦ → L3
Not at all .... 3 → L8

L3 In the past week, have these feelings of panic been:

Running prompt a little uncomfortable or unpleasant 2
or have they been very unpleasant or unbearable? 1

L4 Did this panic/the worst of these panics last for longer than 10 minutes?

Yes 1
No 2

L5 Are you relatively free of anxiety between these panics?

Yes 1
No 2

40

Sr N1364A Apr'94 V5

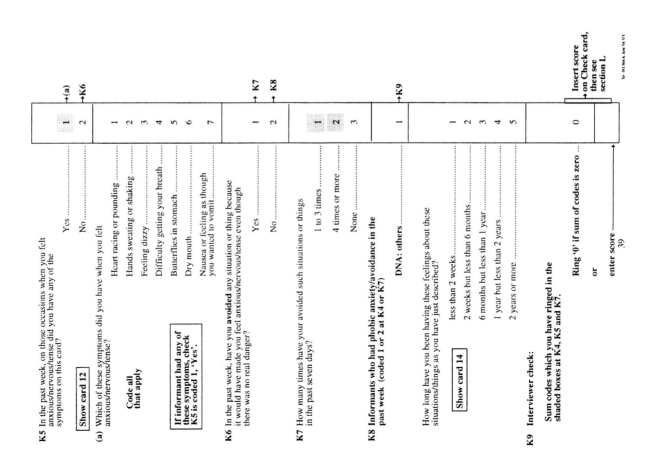

K5 In the past week, on those occasions when you felt anxious/nervous/tense did you have any of the symptoms on this card?

Show card 12

Yes .... 1 → (a)
No .... 2 → K6

(a) Which of these symptoms did you have when you felt anxious/nervous/tense?

Code all that apply

Heart racing or pounding 1
Hands sweating or shaking 2
Feeling dizzy 3
Difficulty getting your breath 4
Butterflies in stomach 5
Dry mouth 6
Nausea or feeling as though you wanted to vomit 7

If informant had any of these symptoms, check K5 is coded 1, 'Yes'.

K6 In the past week, have you **avoided** any situation or thing because it would have made you feel anxious/nervous/tense even though there was no real danger?

Yes .... 1 → K7
No .... 2 → K8

K7 How many times have your avoided such situations or things in the past seven days?

1 to 3 times 1
4 times or more 2
None .... 3 → K9

K8 Informants who had phobic anxiety/avoidance in the past week (coded 1 or 2 at K4 or K7)

DNA: others .... 1 → K9

How long have you been having these feelings about these situations/things as you have just described?

Show card 14

less than 2 weeks 1
2 weeks but less than 6 months 2
6 months but less than 1 year 3
1 year but less than 2 years 4
2 years or more 5

K9 Interviewer check:

Sum codes which you have ringed in the shaded boxes at K4, K5 and K7.

Ring '0' if sum of codes is zero 0
or
enter score ____ → Insert score on Check card, then see section L

39

Sr N1364A Apr'94 V5

L6 Informants who had phobic anxiety

DNA: Others (coded 2 at K1) .... 1 →L7

Refer to situation/thing at K3.

Is this panic always brought on by (SITUATION/THING)?

Yes 1
No 2

L7 How long have you been having these feelings of panic as you have described?

Show card 14

less than 2 weeks 1
2 weeks but less than 6 months 2
6 months but less than 1 year 3
1 year but less than 2 years 4
2 years or more 5

L8 Interviewer check:

Sum codes which you have ringed in the shaded boxes at L2, L3, and L4.

Ring '0' if sum of codes is zero 0

or

enter score ——— →Insert score on Check card, then go to section M

Sr. NI364A Am'94 V5

---

[*] M Compulsions

M1 In the past month, did you find that you kept on doing things over and over again when you knew you had already done them, for instance checking things like taps or washing yourself when you had already done so?

Yes .... 1 →M2
No .... 2 →Go to section N

M2 On how many days in the past week did you find yourself doing things over again that you had already done?

4 days or more .... 1 →M3
1 to 3 days 2
None .... 3 →M9

M3 Since last (DAY OF WEEK) what sorts of things have you done over and over again?

M4 During the past week, have you tried to stop yourself repeating (BEHAVIOUR)/doing any of these things over again?

Yes 1
No 2

M5 Has repeating (BEHAVIOUR)/doing any of these things over again made you upset or annoyed with yourself in the past week?

Yes, upset or annoyed 1
No, not at all 2

Sr. NI364A Am'94 V5

M6 If more than one thing is repeated at M3

DNA : others ...... 1 → M7

Thinking about the past week, which of the things you mentioned did you repeat the **most** times?

Describe here ...... → M7

M7 Since last (DAY OF WEEK), how many times did you repeat (BEHAVIOUR) when you had already done it?

3 or more repeats 1
2 repeats 2
1 repeat 3

Refer to BEHAVIOUR at M6, if applicable

M8 How long have you been repeating (BEHAVIOUR)/any of the things you mentioned in the way which you have described?

Show card 14

less than 2 weeks 1
2 weeks but less than 6 months 2
6 months but less than 1 year 3
1 year but less than 2 years 4
2 years or more 5

M9 Interviewer check:

Sum codes which you have ringed in the shaded boxes at M2, M4, M5 and M7.

Ring '0' if sum of codes is zero 0

or

enter score ____ → **Insert score on Check card, then go to section N**

＊ N Obsessions

N1 In the past month did you have any thoughts or ideas over and over again that you found unpleasant and would prefer not to think about, that still kept on coming into your mind?

Yes ...... 1 → N2
No ...... 2 → **Go to section O**

N2 Can I check, is this the **same** thought or idea over and over again or are you worrying about something in general?

Same thought ...... 1 → N3
Worrying in general ...... 2 → **See instruction below, then go to section O**

Make a note on check flap to go to section I to record this worry, if not already recorded.

N3 What are these unpleasant thoughts or ideas that keep coming into your mind?

Do not probe
Do not press for answer

N4 Since last (DAY OF WEEK), on how many days have you had these unpleasant thoughts?

4 days or more ...... 1 ┐
1 to 3 days ...... 2 → N5
None ...... 3 → N9

N5 During the past week, have you tried to stop yourself thinking any of these thoughts?

Yes 1
No 2

N6 Have you become upset or annoyed with yourself when you have had these thoughts in the past week?

Yes, upset or annoyed 1
Not at all 2

O   Overall effects

Informants who scored 2 or more on any section, A to N.

DNA: Others (All section scores 0 or 1 on check card) ...... 1 → **Complete Check card, then complete front page**

Now I would like to ask you how all of these things that you have told me about have affected you overall.

In the past week, has the way you have been feeling ever actually **stopped** you from getting on with things you used to do or would like to do?

Yes .... 1 → (a)
No .... 2 → (b)

(a) In the past week, has the way you have been feeling stopped you doing things once or more than once?

Once 1
More than once 2
→ **Complete Check card, then complete front page**

(b) Has the way you have been feeling made things more difficult even though you have got everything done?

Yes 1
No 2
→ **Complete Check card, then complete front page**

Sr. N1 94A Apr'94 V

46

N7   In the past week, was the longest episode of having such thoughts :

Running prompt   a quarter of an hour or longer 1
or   was it less than this? 2

N8   How long have you been having these thoughts in the way which you have just described?

Show card 14

less than 2 weeks 1
2 weeks but less than 6 months 2
6 months but less than 1 year 3
1 year but less than 2 years 4
2 years or more 5

N9   Interviewer check:

Sum codes which you have ringed in the shaded boxes at N4, N5, N6 and N7.

Ring '0' if sum of codes is zero ... 0
or
enter score _____ → **Insert score on Check card, then go to section O**

Sr. N1 94A Apr'94 V5

45

N1364

F

Person

Stick serial number label

Check card   **Enter Scores :**

A   Somatic symptoms

B   Fatigue

C   Concentration and forgetfulness

D   Sleep problems

E   Irritability

F   Worry about physical health

G   Depression

H   Depressive ideas

I   Worry

J   Anxiety

K   Phobias

L   Panic

M   Compulsions

N   Obsessions

Total score: sections A to N
→ Enter here

Now complete front page.

Note: Threshold is 12 or more

Se. N1364 Mar '94 V2

N1364

Reference Card A

Auditory hallucinations	Mild schizophrenia
Bipolar affective disorder	Mood swings
Catatonic schizophrenia	Neuroleptic
Chronic schizophrenia	Paranoia
Hallucinations	Paranoid schizophrenia
Hearing voices	Psychosis
Hebephrenic schizophrenia	Psychotic related disorder
Hypomania	Psychotic tendencies
Mania	Schizo-affective disorder
Manic depression	Schizophrenia
Manic depressive psychosis	Schizophrenic affective disorder
Mental illness	Simple schizophrenia
Mentally disturbed	Voices
Mild psychosis	

Reference card B

Anquil	Haldol decanoate	Priadel
Benperidol	Halperidol	Prochloperazine
Camcolit	Largactil	Promazine hydrochloride
Chlorpromazine	Liskonum	Redeptin
Clopixol acuphase	Litarex	Remoxipride
Clopixol	Lithium	Risperdal
Clozapine	Loxapac	Risperidone
Clozaril	Loxapine	Roxiam
Depixol	Melleril	Serenace
Dolmatil	Methotrimeprazine	Sparine
Dozic	Modecate	Stelazine
Droleptan	Moditen	Sulphiride
Droperidol	Moditen ethanate	Sulpiti
Fentazin	Neulactil	Thioridazine
Fluanxol	Nozinan	Trifluoperazine
Flupenthixol	Orap	Trifluperidol
Flupenthixol decanoate	Oxypertine	Zuclopenthixol dihydrochloride
Fluphenazine hydrochloride	Pericyazine	Zuclopenthixol acetate
Fluphenazine decanoate	Perphenazine	Zuclopenthixol decanoate
Fluphenazine enanthate	Phasal decanoate	*Antipsychotic drugs*
Fluspirilene	Pimozide	*Antipsychotic injections*
Fortunan	Piportil	*Depot injections*
Haldol	Pipothiazine palmitate	*Antimanic drugs*

Reference card D

Guide to completing outcome summary before despatch
on front page of A or DN, and recall sheet

Long - standing psychotic illness
rung at 14 (b) [page 6(A) or page 5(DN)] → | 1 ill |

Anti - psychotic medication/injection
rung at 19 [page 8(A) or page 7(DN)] → | 2 med inj |

Doctor stated psychotic illness
rung at 23(b) [page 9 (A) or page 8(DN)] → | 3 Dr |

Screened positive on PSQ
rung at P6 (any of P1 to P5)
[pages 10 to 12 (A) or pages 9 to 11 (DN)] → | 4 PSQ |

Score on check card (00 to 57) ....
[Does not apply in daycentres/nightshelters] → | CIS |

Score on GH self-completion:
total number of ticks in boxes
3 and 4 (range of 00 to 12) .... → | GHQ |

N1364   **Daycentres and Nightshelters Schedule**   **DN**
(No proxies)

IN CONFIDENCE

Stick serial number label

Person   Date of Interview   9   4

Auth no.

Interviewer's Name _ _ _ _ _ _ _ _ _ _

(i) Interviewer code at start of interview

Nightshelter .... 1 → Go to question 1, page 2

Daycentre 2

Code at end of interview

(ii) Type of interview

Full interview, ... 1 → Ask recall

Partial interview 2

Refusal 3

Any question ringed (see pages 5, 7, 8, 9, 10 or 11) .... 1 → Ask recall

Others .... 2 → End interview

(iii) Outcome of sift

(1)

(iv) Interviewer: see reference card D and code before despatch

Outcome summary: Ring all that apply and enter scores

1	2	3	4	
III	med inj	Dr	PRQ	GHQ

→ **Transfer to Recall sheet if anything rung at 1 - 4**

CI-1364DN MAY 94 V9

1

181

7. **Ask or record**

   Where did you sleep last night. I mean did you sleep rough or did you have some accommodation?

Slept rough (include tent)	1	→8
Had accommodation	2	→9
DK/can't remember	3	→8

8. How long is it since you last spent the night in accommodation?

Less than 1 week ago	1
1 week, less than one month ago	2
1 month, less than 3 months ago	3
3 months, less than 6 months ago	4
6 months, less than one year ago	5
1 year or more	6
DK/can't remember	7 →9

   Prompt as necessary

9. In what type of accommodation was that?

   Code one only **Prompt as necessary**

Private accom	
Informants owned/rented house/flat/bedsit	01
Parents home	02
Foster parents	03
Friend/relatives	04
Squat	05
Accommodation provided with job	06
Lodgings/hostel	
Lodgings	07
Bed & Breakfast	08
Hostel/resettlement unit	09
Night shelter	10
Homes	
Children's home	11
Old people's home/sheltered housing	12
Hospitals/medical units	
General hospital	13
Psychiatric unit or hospital	14
Alcohol unit	15
Drug unit	16
Prisons/borstals	
Prison/remand centre/police cell	17
Young offenders institution/detention centre/borstal	18
Other	
Other	19
Dk/can't remember	20

CI:1364DN May'94 V9

3

Demographic details

1. **Sex: Ask or record**

Male	1
Female	2

2. **Age now** ___

3. **Marital status**

Married	1
Cohabiting	2
Single	3
Widowed	4
Divorced/Sep	5

4. To which of the groups listed on this card do you consider you belong?

   Show card 1

White	1
Black - Caribbean	2
Black - African	3
Black - other	4
Indian	5
Pakistani	6
Bangladeshi	7
Chinese	8
None of these	9

Accommodation

5. **Ask or record**

   Can I check, have you slept rough on any of the past seven nights?

Yes (include tent)	1	→7
No	2	→6
DK/can't remember	3	→6

6. **Interviewer check:**

Nightshelter	1	→7
Daycentre	2	End interview (ineligible)

CI:1364DN May'94 V9

2

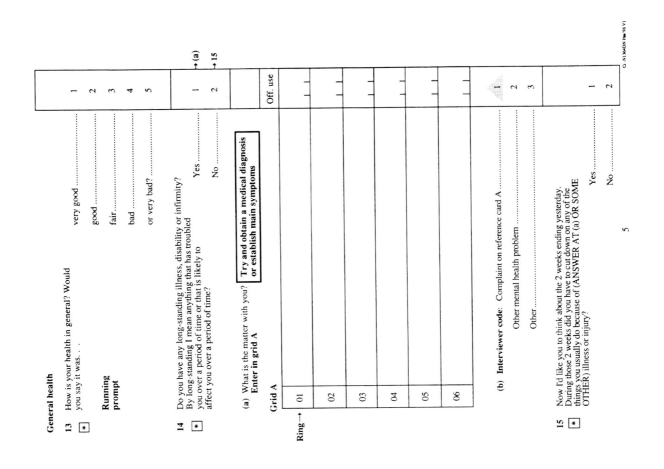

General health

13 How is your health in general? Would you say it was. . .

Running prompt

very good	1
good	2
fair	3
bad	4
or very bad?	5

14 Do you have any long-standing illness, disability or infirmity? By long-standing I mean anything that has troubled you over a period of time or that is likely to affect you over a period of time?

Yes	1	→(a)
No	2	→15

(a) What is the matter with you? **Enter in grid A**

Try and obtain a medical diagnosis or establish main symptoms

Grid A

Ring→

		Off. use
01		
02		
03		
04		
05		
06		

(b) **Interviewer code:**

Complaint on reference card A	1
Other mental health problem	2
Other	3

15 Now I'd like you to think about the 2 weeks ending yesterday. During those 2 weeks did you have to cut down on any of the things you usually do because of (ANSWER AT (a) OR SOME OTHER) illness or injury?

Yes	1
No	2

5

---

10. DNA: not in accommodation for 1 year or more (coded 6 at question 8) .... 1 → Go to 11

In the past 12 months, in total how long would you say you have spent sleeping rough?

Prompt as necessary

Less than 1 week	1
1 week, less than 1 month	2
1 month, less than 6 months	3
6 months or more	4
DK/can't remember	5

11. What sort of place was the last place that you thought of as home?

Current accommodation	21
Never had a 'home'	22

Code one only

Private accom

Informants owned/rented house/flat/bedsit	01
Parents home	02
Foster parents	03
Friend/relatives	04
Squat	05
Accommodation provided with job	06

Prompt as necessary

Lodgings/hostel

Lodgings	07
Bed & Breakfast	08
Hostel/resettlement unit	09
Night shelter	10

Homes

Children's home	11
Old people's home/sheltered housing	12

Hospitals/medical units

General hospital	13
Psychiatric unit or hospital	14
Alcohol unit	15
Drug unit	16

Prisons/borstals

Prison/remand centre/police cell	17
Young offenders institution/detention centre/borstal	18

Other

Other	19
Dk/can't remember	20

12. When were you last living there? DK/can't remember 5

less than 1 week ago	1

Prompt as necessary

1 week, less than 1 month	2
1 month, less than 6 months ago	3
6 months, less than 1 year ago	4

or 1 year or more: enter no. of years

4

183

Grid C

	(b) Ring 1 or 2		Office use
	Taking	Not taking	
1	1	2	
2	1	2	
3	1	2	

Ring →

18 Can I check, are you for some reason **not** taking medicines or having any injections which have been prescribed for you (that you are supposed to be taking)?

Yes .... 1 → (a)
No .... 2 → 19

(a) What is it? (What are they?)

Medication: enter in grid B, page 6 and ring '2' at (b) to indicate 'not taking'

Injection: enter in grid C, above and ring '2' at (b) to indicate 'not taking'

19 Interviewer refer to grids B and C and code:

Medication/injection on reference card B (include if 'not taking') .... 1 → (a)

Others 2

20 If you were feeling unwell, is there a doctor or medical centre you know that you could go to?

Yes 1
No 2
DK 3

(a) Can I check, are you registered with a doctor anywhere?

Yes 1
No 2
Dk/can't remember 3

O-N1364DN/Fas'96 V1

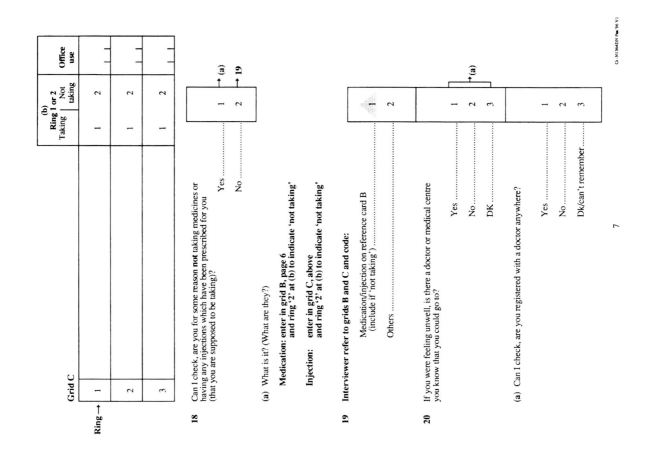

---

16 (May I just check), are you taking any pills or tablets or any other medicine by mouth which have been prescribed for you?

Exclude lotions, ointments, creams, contraceptives

Yes .... 1 → (a)
No .... 2 → 17

(a) What is the name of the pills, tablets or medicine you are taking?

Enter in grid B below, and ring code '1' at (b)

**Try to get brand name or description, or find out what condition it is for.
Ask to look at bottle or box if clarification is required**

Grid B

	(b) Ring 1 or 2		Office use
	Taking	Not taking	
01	1	2	
02	1	2	
03	1	2	
04	1	2	
05	1	2	
06	1	2	
07	1	2	
08	1	2	
09	1	2	

Ring →

17 Are you having a regular course of injections that have been prescribed for you?

Yes .... 1 → (a)
No .... 2 → 18

(a) What is it? (What are they?)
Enter in grid C (opposite) and ring code '1' at (b)

O-N1364DN/Fas'96 V1

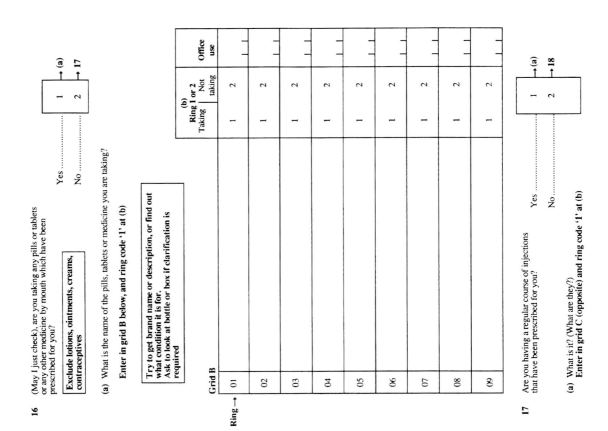

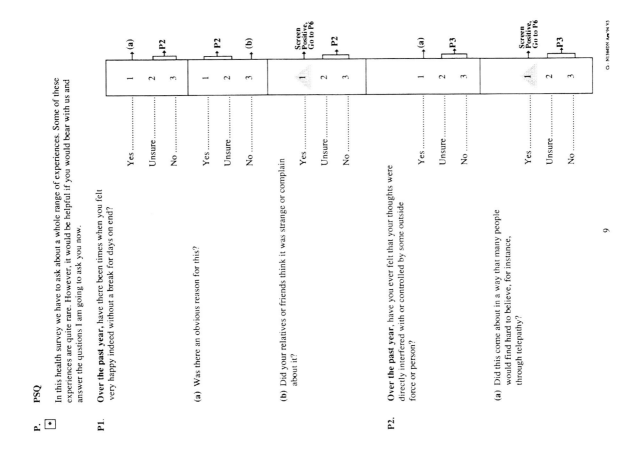

P. PSQ

[*] In this health survey we have to ask about a whole range of experiences. Some of these experiences are quite rare. However, it would be helpful if you would bear with us and answer the questions I am going to ask you now.

P1. **Over the past year**, have there been times when you felt very happy indeed without a break for days on end?

Yes	1	→(a)
Unsure	2	→P2
No	3	

(a) Was there an obvious reason for this?

Yes	1	→P2
Unsure	2	
No	3	→(b)

(b) Did your relatives or friends think it was strange or complain about it?

Yes	1	Screen Positive, Go to P6
Unsure	2	→P2
No	3	

P2. **Over the past year**, have you ever felt that your thoughts were directly interfered with or controlled by some outside force or person?

Yes	1	→(a)
Unsure	2	→P3
No	3	

(a) Did this come about in a way that many people would find hard to believe, for instance, through telepathy?

Yes	1	Screen Positive, Go to P6
Unsure	2	→P3
No	3	

O. N1364DN Apr '94 V5

9

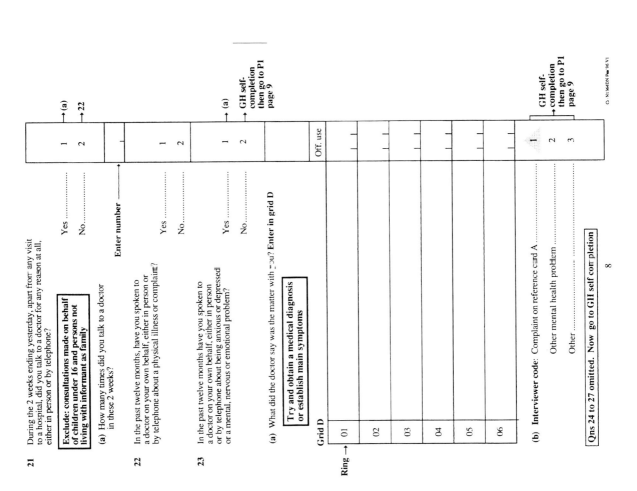

21 During the 2 weeks ending yesterday, apart from any visit to a hospital, did you talk to a doctor for any reason at all, either in person or by telephone?

Exclude: consultations made on behalf of children under 16 and persons not living with informant as family

Yes	1	→(a)
No	2	→22

(a) How many times did you talk to a doctor in these 2 weeks?

Enter number _____

22 In the past twelve months, have you spoken to a doctor on your own behalf, either in person or by telephone about a physical illness or complaint?

Yes	1
No	2

23 In the past twelve months have you spoken to a doctor on your own behalf, either in person or by telephone about being anxious or depressed or a mental, nervous or emotional problem?

Yes	1	→(a)
No	2	GH self-completion then go to P1 page 9

(a) What did the doctor say was the matter with you? **Enter in grid D**

Try and obtain a medical diagnosis or establish main symptoms

Grid D

	Off. use
Ring → 01	
02	
03	
04	
05	
06	

(b) Interviewer code:

Complaint on reference card A	1	GH self-completion then go to P1 page 9
Other mental health problem	2	
Other	3	

Qns 24 to 27 omitted. Now go to GH self completion

8

O. N1364DN Feb '96 V1

185

P3. Over the past year, have there been times when you felt that people were against you?

Yes .... 1 →(a)
Unsure .... 2 →P4
No 3

(a) Have there been times when you felt that people were deliberately acting to harm you or your interests?

Yes .... 1 →(b)
Unsure .... 2 →P4
No 3

(b) Have there been times you felt that a group of people was plotting to cause you serious harm or injury?

Yes .... 1 → Screen Positive, Go to P6
Unsure .... 2 →P4
No 3

P4 Over the past year, have there been times when you felt that something strange was going on?

Yes .... 1 →(a)
Unsure .... 2 →P5
No 3

(a) Did you feel it was so strange that other people would find it very hard to believe?

Yes .... 1 → Screen Positive, Go to P6
Unsure .... 2 →P5
No 3

O - N1360N Am '94 V5

P5. Over the past year, have there been times when you heard or saw things that other people couldn't?

Yes .... 1 →(a)
Unsure .... 2 → Screen Negative, Go to P6
No 3

a) Did you at any time hear voices saying quite a few words or sentences when there was no one around that might account for it?

Yes .... 1 → Screen Positive, Go to P6
Unsure .... 2 → Screen Negative, Go to P6
No 3

P6. Interviewer check

Informant screened positive 1
Informant screened negative 2

Now go to section B, page 12

O - N1360N Am '94 V5

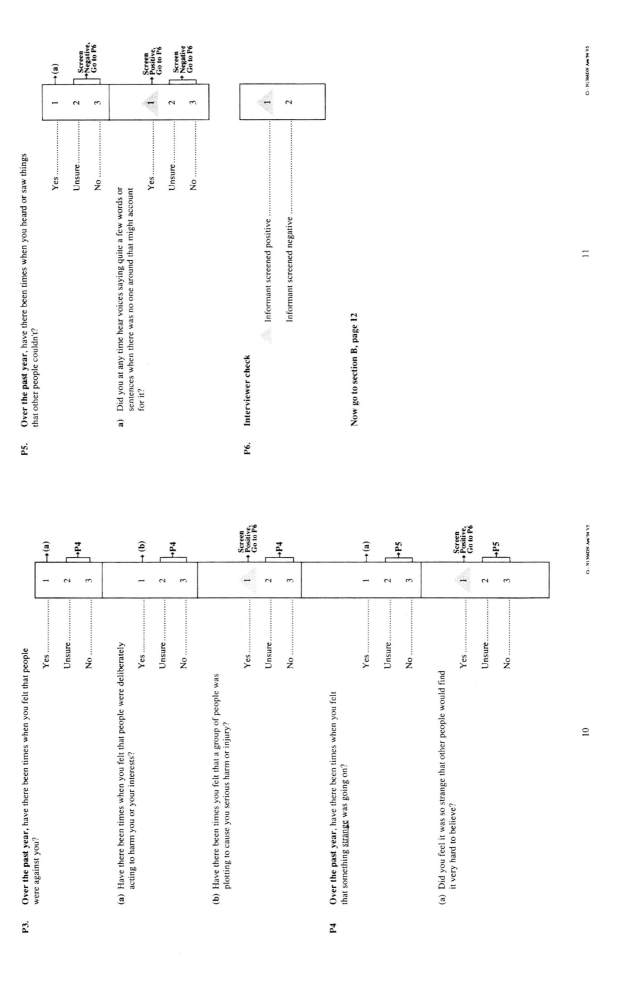

B. Medication and treatment

B1 DNA: No medication or injections (coded 2 at qns.16, 17 and 18, pages 6 and 7) .... 1 →**B2**

Ring column number when appropriate →

(a) Transcribe list of pills, medication or injections from grids on pages 6 and 7.

Include if informant is not taking medicine/injection when supposed to.

(b) What is its/their strength?

If strength of pills not known, describe colour and note what is written on tablet

(c) How many/much are you supposed to have each day?

Enter number of pills/mls/injections per day
OR if less than one a day
Enter number of pills/mls/injections per month
(Less than one per month = **00**)

Spontaneous: Take as needed..............

(d) For what condition do you take them? (For what condition are you supposed to take them?)

Obtain medical diagnosis AND describe main symptoms

(e) How long have you been having this medication? (How long are you supposed to have been having this medication)

Enter number of years
OR if less than 1 year
Enter number of months
(Less than 1 month = **0 0**)

Grid (first page, columns 1–3):

	1	2	3
(a)	Not taking:Ring→ 1	Not taking:Ring→ 1	Not taking:Ring→ 1
	Injection: Ring→ 1	Injection: Ring→ 1	Injection: Ring→ 1
	OFF USE	OFF USE	OFF USE
(b)			
(c)	OFF USE	OFF USE	OFF USE
	1	1	1
(d)			
(e)	OFF USE	OFF USE	OFF USE

12

Grid (second page, columns 4–8):

	4	5	6	7	8
(a)	Not taking:Ring→ 1	Not taking:Ring→ 1	Not taking:Ring→ 1	Not taking:Ring→ 1	Not taking:Ring→ 1
	Injection: Ring→ 1	Injection: Ring→ 1	Injection: Ring→ 1	Injection: Ring→ 1	Injection: Ring→ 1
	OFF USE	OFF USE	OFF USE	OFF USE	OFF USE
(b)					
(c)	OFF USE	OFF USE	OFF USE	OFF USE	OFF USE
	1	1	1	1	1
(d)					
(e)	OFF USE	OFF USE	OFF USE	OFF USE	OFF USE

13

187

Ring column number when appropriate →	1	2	3	4	5	6	7	8
(f) (Can I check,) do you sometimes not take your medication even though you should?								
Yes.........	1 → (g)	1 → (g)	1 → (g)	1 → (g)	1 → (g)	1 → (g)	1 → (g)	1 → (g)
No.........	2 → (i)	2 → (i)	2 → (i)	2 → (i)	2 → (i)	2 → (i)	2 → (i)	2 → (i)
(g) When was the last time this happened?								
Less than 1 week ago	1	1	1	1	1	1	1	1
At least 1 week but less than 1 month ago	2	2	2	2	2	2	2	2
At least 1 month ago	3	3	3	3	3	3	3	3
[*] (h) What was the reason for this? **Prompt as necessary**								
Code all that apply Forgot...	1	1	1	1	1	1	1	1
Didn't need it...	2	2	2	2	2	2	2	2
Don't like to take drugs...	3	3	3	3	3	3	3	3
Side effects...	4	4	4	4	4	4	4	4
Other...	5	5	5	5	5	5	5	5
(i) (Can I check,) do you sometimes take more medication/pills than the stated dose?								
Yes.........	1 → (j)	1 → (j)	1 → (j)	1 → (j)	1 → (j)	1 → (j)	1 → (j)	1 → (j)
No.........	2 → col 2/ B2	2 → col 3/ B2	2 → col 4/ B2	2 → col 5/ B2	2 → col 6/ B2	2 → col 7/ B2	2 → col 8/ B2	2 → B2
(j) When was the last time this happened?								
Less than 1 week ago	1	1	1	1	1	1	1	1
At least 1 week but less than 1 month ago	2	2	2	2	2	2	2	2
At least 1 month ago	3	3	3	3	3	3	3	3
[*] (k) What was the reason for this?								
Code all that apply Needed more to control symptoms...	1	1	1	1	1	1	1	1
Deliberate overdose...	2	2	2	2	2	2	2	2
Other...	3	3	3	3	3	3	3	3

O - N1364DN Am'94 V5

B2

At the moment are you having any counselling or therapy either here or at a doctor's surgery, a health centre, hospital or clinic or anywhere else such as a daycentre?

Yes..... 1 → (a)
No...... 2 → Section C

Ring column no. when appropriate → 1 2 3

(a) What type of counselling or therapy are you having at the moment?

Code from reference card C if possible

INT/OFF USE

(b) How often do you have this counselling/therapy?

Enter no. of treatments per month →
OR if less than one per month
Enter no. of treatments per year →

Spontaneous: when needed.......... 1 1 1

(c) How long have you been having this counselling/therapy?

Enter number of years →
OR if less than 1 year
Enter number of months (less than 1 month = 0 0) →

(d) For what condition are you having this counselling/therapy?

Obtain medical diagnosis AND describe main symptoms

OFF USE

16

CI-1364DN May'94 V6

C Health, social and voluntary care services

GP consultations

C1 During the two weeks ending yesterday, apart from any visit to a hospital, did you talk to a GP or family doctor on your own behalf, either in person or by telephone?

Yes .... 1 → (a)
No .... 2 → C2

(a) How many times have you talked to your GP or family doctor in the past two weeks?

Enter number of times → (b)

Ask (b) to (d) for the last 4 consultations in the past 2 weeks (1 = most recent)

Ring consultation number →	1	2	3	4
(b) When you spoke to the doctor (on....occasion) did you talk about:				
a physical illness or complaint...	1	1	1	1
or about being anxious or depressed, or a mental, nervous or emotional problem?......	2	2	2	2
Spontaneous: Both of these.............	3	3	3	3
(c) At what type of place did you see the doctor?				
Spontaneous: telephoned..........	1	1	1	1
GP surgery/health centre............	1	1	1	1
Daycentre/hostel clinic	2	2	2	2
Other...........	3	3	3	3

17

CI-1364DN May'94 V6

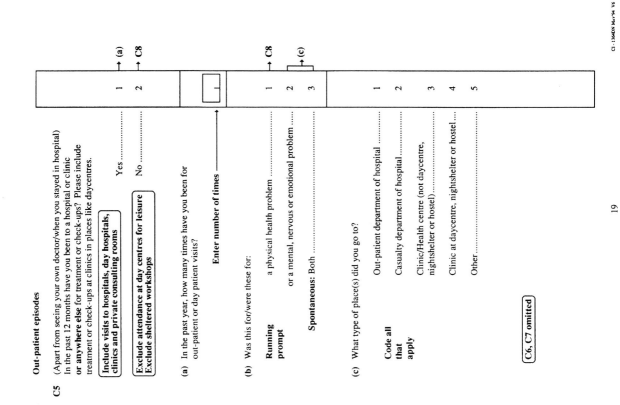

In patient stays

C2 During the past year, that is since (DATE) have you been in hospital or anywhere else as an in-patient, overnight or longer for treatment or tests?

> **Include sight or hearing problems and detoxification**

> **Exclude giving birth**

Yes .... 1 → C3
No .... 2 → C5

C3 In the past 12 months, how many separate stays have you had in hospital or anywhere else as an in-patient?

Enter number of stays ⟶ ☐☐

C4 (In the past year) were you there because of

a physical health problem .... 1 → C5
or a mental nervous or emotional peoblem? 2
Spontaneous: Both .... 3 → (a)

(a) (In the past year) which people did you see when you were in hospital?

> **Show card 2**   **Exclude nurse with non specific duties**

Psychiatrist/Psychotherapist 1
Other consultant or hospital doctor 2
Psychiatric Nurse 3
Social Worker/Counsellor 4
Occupational Therapist 5
Psychologist 6
Voluntary worker 7
Other 8
DK 9

Code all that apply

18

CI - 1364DN May'94 V6

Out-patient episodes

C5 (Apart from seeing your own doctor/when you stayed in hospital) In the past 12 months have you been to a hospital or clinic or **anywhere else** for treatment or check-ups? Please include treatment or check-ups at clinics in places like daycentres.

> **Include visits to hospitals, day hospitals, clinics and private consulting rooms**

> **Exclude attendance at day centres for leisure**
> **Exclude sheltered workshops**

Yes .... 1 → (a)
No .... 2 → C8

(a) In the past year, how many times have you been for out-patient or day patient visits?

Enter number of times ⟶ ☐☐

(b) Was this for/were these for:

Running prompt

a physical health problem .... 1 → C8
or a mental, nervous or emotional problem 2
Spontaneous: Both .... 3 → (c)

(c) What type of place(s) did you go to?

Out-patient department of hospital 1
Casualty department of hospital 2
Clinic/Health centre (not daycentre, nightshelter or hostel) 3
Clinic at daycentre, nightshelter or hostel 4
Other 5

Code all that apply

> **C6, C7 omitted**

19

CI - 1364DN May'94 V6

190

C9 Show card 4

In the past year, have you been offered any help or support from any of the people listed on this card, or indeed any other service, **which you turned down?**

Yes ... 1 →(a)
No ... 2 →C10

(a) What sort of help/service were you offered?

Code all that apply

Community Psychiatric Nurse ... 1
Occupational Therapist/Industrial Therapist ... 2
Social Worker/Counselling Service ... 3
Psychiatrist ... 4
Home care worker/Home help ... 5
Voluntary Worker ... 6
Key worker/care manager ... 7
Other ... 8

(b) Did you turn it down because you did not want or need the help or for some other reason?

* Code all that apply

Did not want/need help ... 1
Could not face it/handle it ... 2
Did not like people/not the right people offering help ... 3
Didn't think it could/would help ... 4
Inconvenient time or location of service ... 5
Did not fit in with housing circumstances ... 6
Other reason ... 7

21

Cl: 1364DN May'94 V6

C8 (Can I check), do you have a key worker?

Yes ... 1 →(a)
No ... 2
Dk ... 3 →(c)

(a) Who is this?

Show card 3

Social worker ... 1
Community Psychiatric Nurse (CPN) ... 2
Occupational Therapist (OT) ... 3
Psychologist ... 4
Psychiatrist ... 5
GP ... 6
Other ... 7

(b) How often do you see the key worker?

Prompt as necessary

At least once a week ... 1
Once a fortnight ... 2
Once a month ... 3
Once every couple of months ... 4
Once or twice a year ... 5
Less than once a year or not at all ... 6

(c) (Can I check), do you have a care manager?

Yes ... 1
No ... 2
Dk ... 3

Note: Care manager may also be the key worker

20

Cl: 1364DN May'94 V6

F Education and Employment Status

F1. At what age did you finish your continuous full-time education at school or college?

Not yet finished 1

Never went to school 2

14 or under 3

15 4

16 5

17 6

18 7

19 or over 8

CI - N1364DN May94 V7

C10 Sometimes people do not see a doctor or other professional about mental, nervous or emotional problems when perhaps they should. In the past year did you decide not to see a doctor or other professional when either you or people around you thought you should?

Yes .... 1 → (a)

No .... 2 → Section F

* **(a)** Thinking about the last time this happened, what were your reasons for not going to a doctor or other professional?

Write verbatim and then code

Code all that apply

Didn't know who to go to or where to go 01

Did not think anyone could help 02

Hour inconvenient/didn't have the time 03

Thought problem would get better by itself 04

Too embarrassed to discuss it with anyone 05

Afraid what family/friends would think 06

Family or friends objected 07

Afraid of consequences (treatment, tests, hospitalisation, sectioned) 08

Afraid of side effects of any treatment 09

Didn't think it was necessary/ No problem 10

A problem one should be able to cope with 11

Other 12

→ Section F

Sections D and E omitted

CI - 1364DN Mar94 V6

Employment status

F3. Did you do any paid work in the last week, that is in the 7 days ending last Sunday, either as an employee or self employed?

| Include paid sheltered employment |
| Include work based training schemes |
| **Exclude college based training schemes** |

Yes .... 01 → F5

No .... → (a)

(a) Even though you weren't working, did you have a job that you were away from last week?

Yes .... 02 → F4

No .... → (i)

(i) Last week were you:

Code first that applies

waiting to take up a job that you had already obtained? 03

looking for work? 04

intending to look for work but prevented by **temporary** ill-health, sickness or injury? 05

going to school or college full time? (use only for persons aged 16 - 49) 06

permanently unable to work because of long term sickness or disability? (for women, use only if aged 16 - 59) 07

retired? (use only if stopped work at age 50 or over) 08

looking after the home or family? 09

or were you doing something else? 10

→ F5

F4. What was the **main** reason you were away from work (last week)?

Code one only

On leave/holiday 1

A mental, nervous or emotional problem 2

A physical health problem 3

Attending a training course away from the workplace 4

Laid off/short time 5

Personal/family reason 6

Problems with housing 7

Other reasons 8

→ F5

25

CI-N1364DN May94 V7

F2. Please look at this card and tell me whether you have passed any of the qualifications listed. Look down the list and tell me the first one you come to that you have passed.

Show card 5

Code first that applies

Degree (or degree level qualification) 1

Teaching qualification
HNC/HND, BEC/TEC Higher, BTEC Higher
City and Guilds Full Technological Certificate 2

Nursing qualifications (SRN, SCM, RGN, RM RHV, Midwife

'A' levels/SCE higher
ONC/OND/BEC/TEC **not** higher
City and Guilds Advanced/Final level 3

'O' level passes (Grade A - C if after 1975)
GCSE (Grades A - C)
CSE Grade 1
SCE Ordinary (Bands A - C)
Standard Grade (Level 1 - 3)
SLC Lower
SUPE Lower or Ordinary
School Certificate or Matric.
City and Guilds Craft/Ordinary level 4

CSE Grades 2 - 5
GCE 'O' level (Grades D & E if after 1975)
GCSE (Grades D, E, F, G)
SCE Ordinary (Bands D & E)
Standard Grade (Level 4, 5)
Clerical or commercial qualifications
Apprenticeship 5

CSE ungraded 6

Other qualifications (**specify**) 7

No qualifications 8

24

F5. Interviewer check

Had a job last week (coded 01 at F3 or 02 at F3(a))	1	→ F8
Unemployed waiting to take up a job (coded 03 at F3(a)(i))	2	→ F6
Unemployed looking for work (coded 04 or 05 at F3(a)(i))	3	→ F7
Others - economically inactive (coded 06 to 10 at F3(a)(i))	4	

F6. Unemployed waiting to take up a job

Apart from the job you are waiting to take up, have you ever had a paid job or done any paid work?

Yes	1	
No	2	→ F8

F7. All others unemployed and economically inactive

(May I check) have you ever had a paid job or done any paid work?

Yes	1	→ F8
No	2	→ See F20, page 30

F8. **If employed**
(i) What was your job last week?

If not employed
(ii) What was your most recent job?

(iii) What is the job you are waiting to take up?

If retired
(iv) What was your main job?

Job title:

Description:

Industry:

SOC	
IND	

F9 (a) **Informant's Definition**

Full-time	1	
Part-time	2	

(b)

Employee	1	→ F9
Self-employed	2	→ F10

F9 (a) **If employee ask or record**

Manager	1
Foreman/supervisor	2
other employee	3

(b) How many employees work(ed) in the establishment

1 - 24	1	
25 - 499	2	→ F11
500 or more	3	

F10 **If self employed**
Do/did you employ other people?

Yes, PROBE: 1 - 24	1
25 - 499	2
500 or more	3
No employees	4

CI - N1364DN May94 V7

F11. **To those with a job last week**

DNA: Unemployed/Economically Inactive
(Coded 2 to 4 at F5, page 26) .... 1 → See F18, page 30

A. For employees (main job/government scheme)
How long have you been with your present employer (up to yesterday)?

Less than 4 weeks 01
4 weeks but less than 3 months 02
3 months but less than 6 months 03
6 months but less than 12 months 04

B. For self-employed (main job)
How long have you been self-employed (up to yesterday)?

Show Card 5(b) and prompt as necessary

12 months but less than 2 years 05
2 years but less than 3 years 06
3 years but less than 5 years 07
5 years but less than 10 years 08
10 years but less than 15 years 09
15 years but less than 20 years 10
20 years but less than 25 years 11
25 years but less than 30 years 12
30 years but less than 35 years 13
35 years but less than 40 years 14
40 years or more 15

F12 omitted

F13. Earlier I was asking you about how you had been feeling in the past month.

Has your health or the way you have been feeling caused you to take time off work in **the past year**?
Yes ..... 1 → (a)
No ..... 2 → F14

(a) How many days in the past year have you taken off work?
Enter number of days →

Weekends falling within a period of sickness must be included

28

F14. **To those with a job last week but temporarily not working because of a mental or physical health problem (coded 2 or 3 at F4, page 25)**   DNA: Others .... 1 → Section G, page 32

How long have you been off work?

Less than 2 weeks 1
2 weeks, less than 1 month 2
1 month, less than 3 months 3
3 months, less than 6 months 4
6 months or more ..... 5 → F16

F15. If employee   DNA: Self-employed (coded 2 at F8(b) page 27). ..... 4 → (a)

Do you expect to return to your present employer?
Yes ..... 1 → F16
No 2
Not sure ..... 3 → F16

(a) Do you expect to return to the same job?
Yes ..... 1 → Section G, page 32
No 2
DK 3

F16. Do you expect to be fit to work again?
Yes ..... 1 → F17
No ..... 2 → Section G, page 32
Not sure 3

F17. Will you look for another paid job in the future?
Yes ..... 1 → Section G, page 32
No ..... 2 → (a)
DK 3

(a) Why will/may you not look for another job?
Code all that apply
No suitable jobs: general employment situation 1
No suitable jobs: due to health problems 2
Too old ..... 3 → Section G, page 32
Housing circumstances make it difficult/impossible 4
Other (specify) 5

29

195

Left form (page 30)

F18. If not working but has worked

DNA: Never worked (code 2 at F6, page 26) .... 1 → See F20

How old were you when you left your last paid job?

Enter age ——→

[F19 omitted]

F20. Interviewer check:

Code first that applies
- Retired (code 08 at F3(a)(vi), page 25). .... 1 → Section G, page 32
- Wating to take up a job (code 2 at F5, page 26) .... 2 → (a)
- Others .... 3 → (b)

If not working but not retired

Is the reason that you are not working at present because ...

Individual prompt
- the way you have been feeling makes it impossible for you to do any kind of paid work? .... 1 → (b)

Code first that applies
- a physical health problem makes it impossible for you to do any kind of paid work? .... 2 → F21
- you have not found a suitable paid job? .... 3 → F21
- your housing circumstances make it difficult for you to keep a paid job? .... 4 → Section G, page 32
- or because you do not want or need a paid job? .... 5 → F21
- Other (specify) .... 6 → F21

(b) May I just check, would you be able to do some kind of sheltered or part-time work if it were available, or is this impossible?

[Priority: code 2]
- Could do sheltered work .... 1 → F21
- Could do part-time work .... 2 → F21
- Impossible to do work .... 3 → Section G, page 32

30

Right form (page 31)

F21. (May I just check) Are you looking for a job at the moment?
- Yes .... 1 → F23
- No .... 2 → (a)

[*] (a) Have you looked for a job at all (since you last worked)?
- Yes .... 1 → F22
- No .... 2 → (i)

[*] (i) Why have you not looked for a job?

Code all that apply
- No suitable jobs around - general employment situation 1
- No suitable jobs for someone with subject's health problem 2
- your housing circumstances make it difficult/impossible to get a paid job? 3
- Other (specify) 4

→ Section G

F22. Why have you stopped looking for jobs?

[*] Code all that apply
- No suitable jobs around - general employment situation 1
- No suitable jobs for someone with subject's health problem 2
- your housing circumstances make it difficult/impossible to get a paid job? 3
- Other (specify) 4

F23. Have you ever/since you last worked done any of the following to help get a job:

Individual prompt

	Yes	No
Visited a local Job Centre?	1	2
Talked to a Careers Officer?	1	2
Talked to a Disablement Resettlement Officer (DRO)?	1	2

[F24 and F25 omitted]

31

196

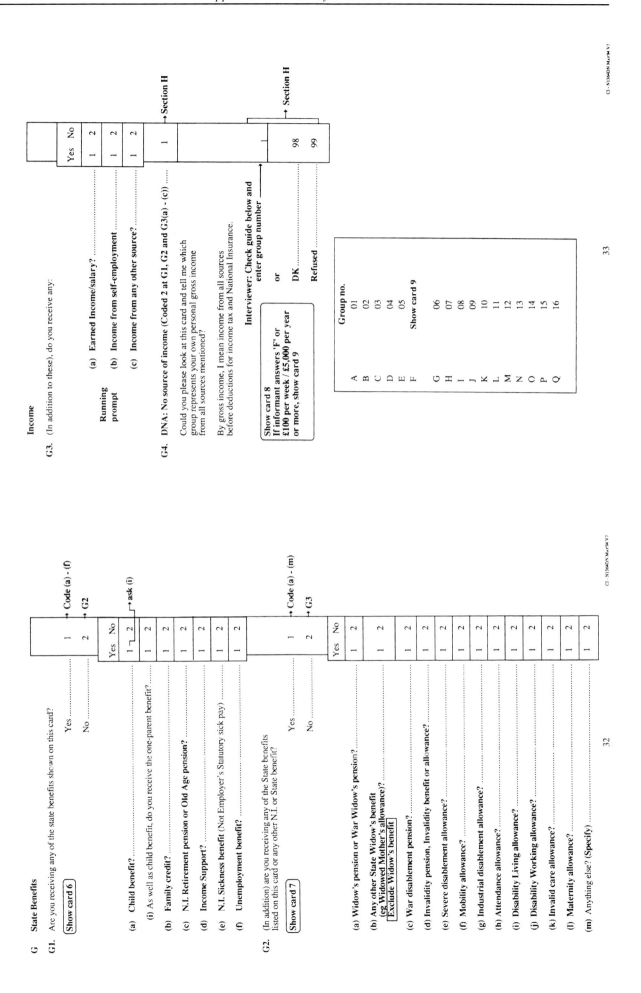

Income

G3. (In addition to these), do you receive any:

		Yes	No	
(a)	**Earned Income/salary?**	1	2	
Running prompt	(b) **Income from self-employment**	1	2	
	(c) **Income from any other source?**	1	2	
		1		→ **Section H**

G4. DNA: No source of income (Coded 2 at G1, G2 and G3(a) - (c)) ......

Could you please look at this card and tell me which group represents your own personal gross income from all sources mentioned?

By gross income, I mean income from all sources before deductions for income tax and National Insurance.

Interviewer: Check guide below and enter group number ———→

Show card 8
If informant answers 'F' or £100 per week / £5,000 per year or more, show card 9

or	
DK	98
Refused	99

→ **Section H**

	Group no.
A	01
B	02
C	03
D	04
E	05
F	**Show card 9**
G	06
H	07
I	08
J	09
K	10
L	11
M	12
N	13
O	14
P	15
Q	16

CI- N1364DN M«r94 V7

33

G State Benefits

G1. Are you receiving any of the state benefits shown on this card?

Show card 6

	Yes	1	→ Code (a) - (f)
	No	2	→ G2

		Yes	No	
(a)	**Child benefit?**	1	2	→ **ask (i)**
	(i) As well as child benefit, do you receive the one-parent benefit?			
(b)	**Family credit?**	1	2	
(c)	**N.I. Retirement pension or Old Age pension?**	1	2	
(d)	**Income Support?**	1	2	
(e)	**N.I. Sickness benefit** (Not Employer's Statutory sick pay)	1	2	
(f)	**Unemployment benefit?**	1	2	

G2. (In addition) are you receiving any of the State benefits listed on this card or any other N.I. or State benefit?

Show card 7

	Yes	1	→ Code (a) - (m)
	No	2	→ G3

		Yes	No
(a)	**Widow's pension or War Widow's pension?**	1	2
(b)	**Any other State Widow's benefit** (eg **Widowed Mother's allowance**)? **Exclude Widow's benefit**	1	2
(c)	**War disablement pension?**	1	2
(d)	**Invalidity pension, Invalidity benefit or allowance?**	1	2
(e)	**Severe disablement allowance?**	1	2
(f)	**Mobility allowance?**	1	2
(g)	**Industrial disablement allowance?**	1	2
(h)	**Attendance allowance?**	1	2
(i)	**Disability Living allowance?**	1	2
(j)	**Disability Working allowance?**	1	2
(k)	**Invalid care allowance?**	1	2
(l)	**Maternity allowance?**	1	2
(m)	**Anything else? (Specify)**	1	2

CI- N1364DN M«r94 V7

32

H Smoking

H1. Have you ever smoked a cigarette, a cigar, or a pipe?

Yes.... 1 → **H2**
No.... 2 → **Go to Section I**

H2. Do you smoke cigarettes at all nowadays?

Yes.... 1 → **(a)**
No.... 2 → **Go to Section I**

(a) About how many cigarettes **a day** do you usually smoke?

Spontaneous: different at weekend/weekday.... 1 → **H3**

Less than 1.... 00 → **Go to Section I**

No. smoked a day ___

H3. About how many cigarettes **a day** do you usually smoke at weekends?

Less than 1.... 00

No. smoked a day ___

H4. And about how many cigarettes **a day** do you usually smoke on weekdays?

Less than 1.... 00

No. smoked a day ___

I Drinking

I1. I'm now going to ask you a few questions about what you drink - that is, if you do drink.

Do you ever drink alcohol nowadays, including drinks you brew or make at home?

Yes.... 1 → **I5**
No.... 2 → **I2**

I2. Could I just check, does that mean you never have an alcoholic drink nowadays, or do you have an alcoholic drink very occasionally, perhaps for medicinal purposes or on special occasions like Christmas or New Year?

Very occasionally.... 1 → **I5**
Never.... 2 → **I3**

I3. Have you always been a non-drinker, or did you stop drinking for some reason?

Always a non-drinker.... 1 → **I4(a)**
Used to drink but stopped.... 2 → **I4(b)**

I4(a). **Always a non drinker**

[*] Why is that?

Code all that apply

Religious reasons.... 1
Don't like it.... 2
Parent's advice.... 3
Health reasons.... 4
Can't afford it.... 5
Other.... 6

Go to page 4, Schedule D, then complete front page

I4(b). **Used to drink but stopped**

[*] What would you say was the main reason you stopped drinking?

Code all that apply

Religious reasons.... 1
Don't like it.... 2
Parent's advice.... 3
Health reasons.... 4
Can't afford it.... 5
Other.... 6

Go to page 4, Schedule D, then complete front page

I5. I'm going to read out a few descriptions about the amounts of alcohol people drink, and I'd like you to say which one fits you best. Would you say you:

[*] **Running prompt**

hardly drink at all.... 1
drink a little.... 2
drink a moderate amount.... 3
drink quite a lot.... 4
or drink heavily?.... 5 → **I6**
DK.... 6

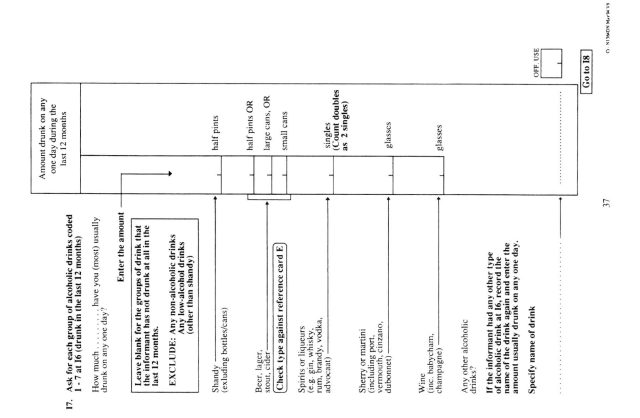

I7. Ask for each group of alcoholic drinks coded 1 - 7 at I6 (drunk in the last 12 months)

How much .... have you (most) usually drunk on any one day?

Enter the amount

Leave blank for the groups of drink that the informant has not drunk at all in the last 12 months.

EXCLUDE: Any non-alcoholic drinks
Any low-alcohol drinks (other than shandy)

	Amount drunk on any one day during the last 12 months
Shandy (excluding bottles/cans)	half pints
Beer, lager, stout, cider	half pints OR / large cans, OR / small cans
Check type against reference card E	
Spirits or liqueurs (e.g. gin, whisky, rum, brandy, vodka, advocaat)	singles (Count doubles as 2 singles)
Sherry or martini (including port, vermouth, cinzano, dubonnet)	glasses
Wine (inc. babycham, champagne)	glasses

Any other alcoholic drinks?

If the informant had any other type of alcoholic drink at I6, record the name of the drink again and enter the amount usually drunk on any one day.

Specify name of drink

Go to I8

OFF. USE

37

O. N136DN May'94 V9

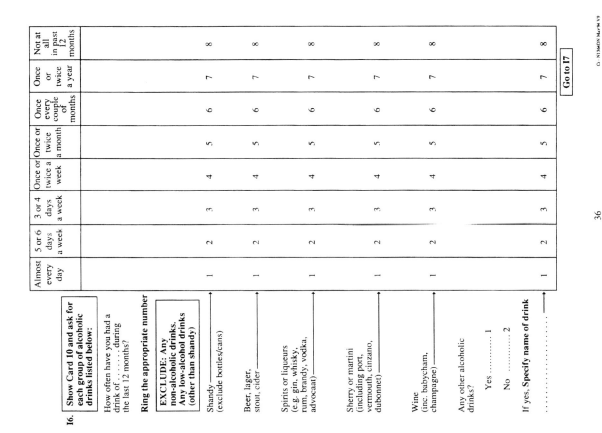

I6. Show Card 10 and ask for each group of alcoholic drinks listed below:

How often have you had a drink of .... during the last 12 months?

Ring the appropriate number

EXCLUDE: Any non-alcoholic drinks. Any low-alcohol drinks (other than shandy)

	Almost every day	5 or 6 days a week	3 or 4 days a week	Once or twice a week	Once or twice a month	Once every couple of months	Once or twice a year	Not at all in past 12 months
Shandy (exclude bottles/cans)	1	2	3	4	5	6	7	8
Beer, lager, stout, cider	1	2	3	4	5	6	7	8
Spirits or liqueurs (e.g. gin, whisky, rum, brandy, vodka, advocaat)	1	2	3	4	5	6	7	8
Sherry or martini (including port, vermouth, cinzano, dubonnet)	1	2	3	4	5	6	7	8
Wine (inc. babycham, champagne)	1	2	3	4	5	6	7	8
Any other alcoholic drinks? Yes ...... 1 No 2								
If yes, Specify name of drink	1	2	3	4	5	6	7	8

Go to I7

36

O. N136DN May'94 V9

I8. During the past year, how often did you have 12 or more **units** of alcoholic drink of any kind in a single day, that is any combination of beers, glasses of wine, or other alcoholic drinks?

This card will help you to work out the number of units.

Show card 10 and use cards 11 and 12 as necessary

Almost every day	1	Go to Schedule D, then complete front page
5 - 6 days a week	2	
3 - 4 days a week	3	
Once or twice a week	4	
Once or twice a month	5	
Once every couple of months	6	
Once or twice a year	7	
Not at all in the past 12 months	8	→ I9

I9. During the past year, how often did you have from 8 to 11 **units** of alcoholic drink of any kind in a single day, that is any combination of beers, glasses of wine, or other alcoholic drinks?

Show card 10 and use cards 11 and 12 as necessary

Almost every day	1	Go to Schedule D, then complete front page
5 - 6 days a week	2	
3 - 4 days a week	3	
Once or twice a week	4	
Once or twice a month	5	
Once every couple of months	6	
Once or twice a year	7	
Not at all in the past 12 months	8	→ I10

I10. During the past year, how often did you have from 5 to 7 **units** of alcoholic drink of any kind in a single day, (that is any combination of beers, glasses of wine, or other alcoholic drinks)?

Show card 10 and use cards 11 and 12 as necessary

Almost every day	1	Go to Schedule D, then complete front page
5 - 6 days a week	2	
3 - 4 days a week	3	
Once or twice a week	4	
Once or twice a month	5	Go to page 4 Schedule D, then complete front page
Once every couple of months	6	
Once or twice a year	7	
Not at all in the past 12 months	8	

O. N136DN May94 V9

N1364   Yellow Schedule   B
               Hostels and PSL

IN CONFIDENCE

Stick serial number label

Person [ ]   Date of Interview   9 | 4

(1)

Complete at end of interview.

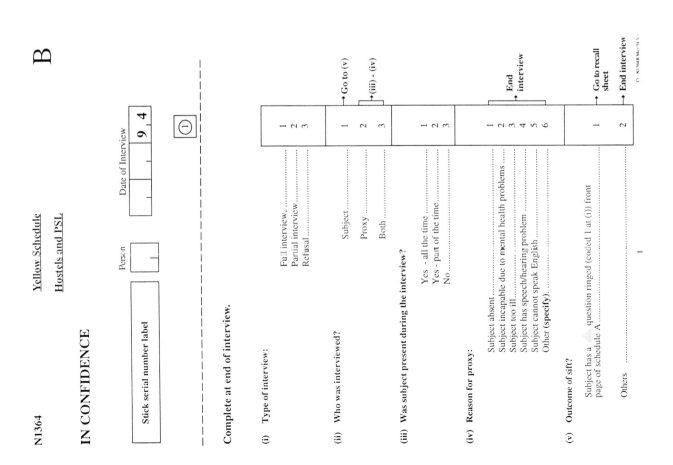

(i) **Type of interview:**

Full interview 1
Partial interview 2
Refusal .... 3 → **Go to (v)**

(ii) **Who was interviewed?**

Subject 1
Proxy .... 2 → **(iii) - (iv)**
Both 3

(iii) **Was subject present during the interview?**

Yes - all the time 1
Yes - part of the time 2
No 3

(iv) **Reason for proxy:**

Subject absent 1
Subject incapable due to mental health problems 2
Subject too ill 3
Subject has speech/hearing problem 4
Subject cannot speak English .... 5 → **End interview**
Other (**specify**) 6

(v) **Outcome of sift?**

Subject has a ▨ question ringed (coded 1 at (i)) front
page of schedule A .... 1 → **Go to recall sheet**

Others .... 2 → **End interview**

201

A   Long-standing illness

A1   Informant has long-standing illness or saw a GP about a mental, nervous or emotional problem

DNA: Informants coded 2 at qn.14, page 6 <u>and</u> at qn.23, page 9, Schedule A .... 1 → **Go to Section B page 4**

Refer to complaints in Schedule A:
See qn.14 (a), page 6 <u>and</u> qn.23 (a), page 9

Earlier you told me about (COMPLAINT(s)).
I'd now like to ask you a few more questions about this.

Transcribe details of complaint(s) from Schedule A.

COMPLAINT No. →	1	2	3	4	5	6	7	8
(a) Name of complaint or Describe main symptoms [Try and obtain medical diagnosis]	OFF USE	OFF USE	OFF USE	OFF USE	OFF USE	OFF USE	OFF USE	OFF USE
(b) How old were you when your (COMPLAINT) started? Enter AGE → [Code 00 if from birth Code 99 if DK]	☐☐	☐☐	☐☐	☐☐	☐☐	☐☐	☐☐	☐☐
(c) For how long has your (COMPLAINT) been at its present level? Enter no. of years OR if less than 1 year Enter no. of months → (less than 1 month = 00)	☐☐ ☐☐	☐☐ ☐☐	☐☐ ☐☐	☐☐ ☐☐	☐☐ ☐☐	☐☐ ☐☐	☐☐ ☐☐	☐☐ ☐☐
(d) In the past week, did your (COMPLAINT) actually stop you from getting on with the things you usually do or would like to do? [*] Yes...... No......	1 2	1 2	1 2	1 2	1 2	1 2	1 2	1 2

G · N136·B Ma·'94·V9

2

3

B. Medication and treatment

B1 DNA: No medication or injections (coded 2 at qns.16, 17 and 18, pages 7 and 8 Schedule A) .... $\boxed{1}$ → B2

Ring column number when appropriate →

	1	2	3	4	5	6	7	8
	Not taking:Ring→ 1	Not taking:Ring→ 1	Not taking:Ring→ 1	Not taking:Ring→ 1	Not taking:Ring→ 1	Not taking:Ring→ 1	Not taking:Ring→ 1	Not taking:Ring→ 1

(a) Transcribe list of pills, medication or injections from grids Band C on pages 7 & 8 Schedule A

Include if informant is not taking medicine/injection when supposed to.

Injection: Ring→ 1	Injection: Ring→ 1	Injection: Ring→ 1	Injection: Ring→ 1	Injection: Ring→ 1	Injection: Ring→ 1	Injection: Ring→ 1	Injection: Ring→ 1
OFF USE	OFF USE	OFF USE	OFF USE	OFF USE	OFF USE	OFF USE	OFF USE

(b) What is its/their strength?

If strength of pills not known, describe colour and note what is written on tablet

OFF USE	OFF USE	OFF USE	OFF USE	OFF USE	OFF USE	OFF USE	OFF USE

(c) How many/much are you supposed to have each day?

Enter number of pills/mls/injections per day →

OR if less than 1 one a day

Enter number of pills/mls/injections per month →

(Less than one per month = 00)

Spontaneous: Take as needed.............

(d) For what condition do you take them? (For what condition are you supposed to take them?)

Obtain medical diagnosis AND describe main symptoms

OFF USE	OFF USE	OFF USE	OFF USE	OFF USE	OFF USE	OFF USE	OFF USE

(e) How long have you been having this medication? (How long are you supposed to have been having this medication)

Enter number of years →

OR if less than 1 year

Enter number of months → (Less than 1 month = 0 0)

G - N1366B Ma-94 V9

4   5

Ring column number when appropriate→	1	2	3	4	5	6	7	8
(f) (Can I check,) do you sometimes not take your medication even though you should?								
Yes......	1 → (g)	1 → (g)	1 → (g)	1 → (g)	1 → (g)	1 → (g)	1 → (g)	1 → (g)
No......	2 → (i)	2 → (i)	2 → (i)	2 → (i)	2 → (i)	2 → (i)	2 → (i)	2 → (i)
(g) When was the last time this happened?								
Less than 1 week ago	1	1	1	1	1	1	1	1
Prompt as necessary — At least 1 week but less than 1 month ago	2	2	2	2	2	2	2	2
At least 1 month ago	3	3	3	3	3	3	3	3
(h) What was the reason for this?								
Code all that apply — Forgot	1	1	1	1	1	1	1	1
Didn't need it	2	2	2	2	2	2	2	2
Don't like to take drugs	3	3	3	3	3	3	3	3
Side effects	4	4	4	4	4	4	4	4
Other	5	5	5	5	5	5	5	5
(i) (Can I check,) do you sometimes take more medication/pills than the stated dose?								
Yes......	1 → (j)	1 → (j)	1 → (j)	1 → (j)	1 → (j)	1 → (j)	1 → (j)	1 → (j)
No......	2 → (l)	2 → (l)	2 → (l)	2 → (l)	2 → (l)	2 → (l)	2 → (l)	2 → (l)
(j) When was the last time this happened?								
Less than 1 week ago	1	1	1	1	1	1	1	1
Prompt as necessary — At least 1 week but less than 1 month ago	2	2	2	2	2	2	2	2
At least 1 month ago	3	3	3	3	3	3	3	3
(k) What was the reason for this?								
Code all that apply — Needed more to control symptoms	1	1	1	1	1	1	1	1
Deliberate overdose	2	2	2	2	2	2	2	2
Other	3	3	3	3	3	3	3	3

G N1364B Mar94 V9

Ring column number when appropriate →	1	2	3	4	5	6	7	8
(l) Transcribe condition from (d), pages 4 and 5.............								
(m) DNA: already asked about this condition in a previous column	X	1 → col 3 or B2	1 → col 4 or B2	1 → col 5 or B2	1 → col 6 or B2	1 → col 7 or B2	1 → col 8 or B2	1 → B2
Have you had any other medication or treatment for (CONDITION AT (l)) which you don't have now Yes	1 → (n)	1 → (n)	1 → (n)	1 → (n)	1 → (n)	1 → (n)	1 → (n)	1 → (n)
No........	2 → (p)	2 → (p)	2 → (p)	2 → (p)	2 → (p)	2 → (p)	2 → (p)	2 → (p)
(n) Did you stop this treatment on your own accord or on professional advice? Own accord.........	1 → (o)	1 → (o)	1 → (o)	1 → (o)	1 → (o)	1 → (o)	1 → (o)	1 → (o)
Professional advice.	2 → (p)	2 → (p)	2 → (p)	2 → (p)	2 → (p)	2 → (p)	2 → (p)	2 → (p)
✱ (o) What made you decide to stop this treatment? Code all that apply Did not work/were not strong enough.........	1	1	1	1	1	1	1	1
Side effects.........	2	2	2	2	2	2	2	2
Other.........	3	3	3	3	3	3	3	3
(p) Have you ever been offered any other medication or treatment for (CONDITION) which you refused? Yes.........	1 → (q)	1 → (q)	1 → (q)	1 → (q)	1 → (q)	1 → (q)	1 → (q)	1 → (q)
No.........	2 → col 2 or B2	2 → col 3 or B2	2 → col 4 or B2	2 → col 5 or B2	2 → col 6 or B2	2 → col 7 or B2	2 → col 8 or B2	2 → B2
(q) What was it?	INT/ OFF USE	INT/ OFF USE	INT/ OFF USE	INT/ OFF USE	INT/ OFF USE	INT/ OFF USE	INT/ OFF USE	INT/ OFF USE
[If treatment, code from reference card C if possible]								
✱ (r) Why did you refuse it? Code all that apply Worry about side effects.........	1	1	1	1	1	1	1	1
Don't like medication/treatment.........	2	2	2	2	2	2	2	2
Other.........	3	3	3	3	3	3	3	3

O: N1364B May'94 V9

8

O: N1364B May'94 V9

9

(page 11)

Ring column number when appropriate →

	1	2	3
(f) DNA: Already asked about this condition in a previous column.... Have you had any other treatment or medication for (CONDITION AT d) which you don't have now? Yes...... No......	✗	1 → col 3 or C1	1 → C1
(g) Did you stop this treatment on your own accord or on professional advice? On own accord...... Professional advice....	1 → (g) 2 → (i)	1 → (g) 2 → (i)	1 → (g) 2 → (i)
	1 → (h) 2 → (i)	1 → (h) 2 → (i)	1 → (h) 2 → (i)
(h) What made you decide to stop this treatment? Code all that apply — Did not work/was not strong enough...... Side effects...... Other......	1 2 3	1 2 3	1 2 3
(i) Have you ever been offered any other treatment or medication for (CONDITION AT d) which you refused? Yes...... No......	1 → (j) 2 → col 2 or C1	1 → (j) 2 → col 3 or C1	1 → (j) 2 → C1
(j) What was it?			
(k) Why did you refuse it? Code all that apply — Worry about side effects...... Don't like medication/treatment...... Other......	INT/ OFF USE 1 2 3	INT/ OFF USE 1 2 3	INT/ OFF USE 1 2 3

O. N1356B May '94 V9

11

(page 10)

B2 At the moment are you having any counselling or therapy either here or at a doctor's surgery, a health centre, hospital or clinic or anywhere else such as a daycentre? →

Yes...... 1 → (a)
No...... 2 → Section C page 12

Ring column no. when appropriate →

	1	2	3
(a) What type of counselling or therapy are you having at the moment? Code from reference card C if possible			
(b) How often do you have this counselling/therapy? Enter no. of treatments per month → OR if less than one per month Enter no. of treatments per year → Spontaneous: when needed.........	INT/ OFF USE	INT/ OFF USE	INT/ OFF USE
(c) How long have you been having this counselling/therapy? Enter number of years → OR if less than 1 year Enter number of months → (less than 1 month = 0 0)			
(d) For what condition are you having this counselling/therapy? Obtain medical diagnosis AND describe main symptoms			
(e) Interviewer check: Is condition at B2(d) mentioned at B1(d), pages 4 and 5? Yes...... No......	OFF USE 1 → col 2 or C1 2 → (f)	OFF USE 1 → col 3 or C1 2 → (f)	OFF USE 1 → C1 2 → (f)

O. N1356B May '94 V9

10

206

Blank page

13

C   Health, social and voluntary care services

GP consultations

C1 During the two weeks ending yesterday, apart from any visit to a hospital, did you talk to a GP or family doctor on your own behalf, either in person or by telephone?

Yes .... 1 → (a)

No .... 2 → C2

(a) How many times have you talked to your GP or family doctor in the past two weeks?

Enter number of times → (b)

Ask (b) to (d) for the last 4 consultations (1 = most recent)

Ring consultation number →	1	2	3	4
(b) When you spoke to the doctor (on....occasion) did you talk about:				
a physical illness or complaint..	1	1	1	1
Running prompt or about being anxious or depressed, or a mental, nervous or emotional problem?........	2	2	2	2
Spontaneous: Both of these..........	3	3	3	3
(c) Were you satisfied or dissatisfied with the consultation?				
Satisfied..........	1→col 2 or C2	1→col 3 or C2	1→col 4 or C2	1→C2
Dissatisfied..........	2→(d)	2→(d)	2→(d)	2→(d)
(d) In what way were you dissatisfied?				
Doctor does not listen, not interested, ignores me..........	1	1	1	1
Informant thinks treatment was inappropriate..........	2	2	2	2
Code all that apply Informant not given tests, treatment or hospitalisation...	3	3	3	3
Doctor said there was nothing wrong or nothing s/he could do...	4	4	4	4
Other..........	5	5	5	5

12

In patient stays

C2 During the past year, that is since (DATE) have you been in hospital or anywhere else as an in-patient, overnight or longer for treatment or tests?

[Include sight or hearing problems and detoxification]

[Exclude giving birth]

Yes	1 →C3
No	2 →C5, page 16

C3 In the past 12 months, how many separate stays have you had in hospital or anywhere else as an in-patient?

Enter number of stays →

C4 Ask (a) to (d) for the last 4 in-patient episodes (1=most recent)

Ring in-patient episode number →	1	2	3	4
(a) How many nights altogether were you there on the (.....) stay? Enter number of nights →				
(b) Were you there because of				
Running prompt — a physical health problem	1→col 2 or C5	1→col 3 or C5	1→col 4 or C5	1→C5
or a mental nervous or emotional problem?	2 ⌐(c)⌐ 3	2 ⌐(c)⌐ 3	2 ⌐(c)⌐ 3	2 ⌐(c)⌐ 3
Spontaneous: Both				

Ring in-patient episode number →	1	2	3	4
(c) Who referred you to hospital?				
GP	01	01	01	01
Community Psychiatric Nurse	02	02	02	02
Social worker	03	03	03	03
Psychiatrist	04	04	04	04
Via casualty (A and E)	05	05	05	05
Via law courts/Probation Service or Police	06	06	06	06
Self-admitted	07	07	07	07
Key worker/Care manager	08	08	08	08
Other	09	09	09	09
(d) When you were there which people did you see? [Show card 15] [Exclude nurse with non specific duties]				
Code all that apply — Psychiatrist/Psychotherapist	01	01	01	01
Other consultant or hospital doctor	02	02	02	02
Psychiatric Nurse	03	03	03	03
Social Worker/Counsellor	04	04	04	04
Occupational Therapist (OT)	05	05	05	05
Psychologist	06	06	06	06
Voluntary worker	07	07	07	07
Other	08	08	08	08

Out-patient episodes

C5 (Apart from seeing your own doctor/when you stayed in hospital) In the past 12 months have you been to a hospital or clinic **or anywhere else** for treatment or check-ups? Please include treatment or check-ups at clinics in places like daycentres.

[Include visits to hospitals, day hospitals, clinics and private consulting rooms]

[**Exclude attendance at day centres for leisure. Exclude sheltered workshops**]

Yes .... 1 →(a)
No .... 2 → C7, page 18

(a) How many different places have you been for out-patient or day patient visits in the past year?

Enter number of places →

C6 For each place attended, ring column number and ask (a) to (f)

Ring column no. →	1	2	3	4
(a) Was your outpatient or day patient visit because of a physical health problem ...	1 → col 2 or C7	1 → col 3 or C7	1 → col 4 or C7	1 → C7
Running prompt or a mental, nervous or emotional problem? ... *Spontaneous* - Both ...	2 ⌐(b) 3	2 ⌐(b) 3	2 ⌐(b) 3	2 ⌐(b) 3
(b) What type of place did you go to?				
Out-patient dept. of hospital ...	1	1	1	1
Casualty dept. of hospital ...	2	2	2	2
Clinic/Health Centre (not daycentre/hostel) ...	3	3	3	3
Private consulting rooms ...	4	4	4	4
Day centre/Hostel clinic ...	5	5	5	5
Other ...	6	6	6	6
(c) How many times have you been to the (PLACE) in the past year? Enter no. of times →	☐	☐	☐	☐

Ring column no. when appropriate →

C6(d) Which of these people did you normally see at this hospital/clinic?

[**Exclude nurse with non specific duties**]

Show card 16

Code all that apply

	1	2	3	4
Psychiatrist/Psychotherapist ...	01	01	01	01
Other consultant/hospital doctor ...	02	02	02	02
Psychiatric Nurse ...	03	03	03	03
Social worker/Counsellor ...	04	04	04	04
Occupational Therapist (OT) ...	05	05	05	05
Psychologist ...	06	06	06	06
Other ...	07	07	07	07
(e) Are you currently attending (PLACE)? Yes ...	1→ col 2 or C7	1→ col 3 or C7	1→ col 4 or C7	1→ C7
No ...	2 → (f)	2 → (f)	2 → (f)	2 → (f)
(f) Have you stopped going of your own accord or were you discharged? On own accord ...	1	1	1	1
Discharged ...	2	2	2	2
Spontaneous Haven't stopped going, go as needed ...	3	3	3	3

C7 Here is a list of people who visit people where they live/ are staying to give them help and support when they need it. In the past year have any of these people visited you?

Yes.......... 1 → (a)

No .... 2 → C8, page 20

PSL: Show card 17
Hostel: Show card 18

**Ring person no.
Code all that apply →**

	Community Psychiatric Nurse	Occupational Therapist	Social Worker	Psychiatrist	Home care worker/ Home help	PSL only DNA: Hostels (go to C8)	
						Voluntary Worker	Second Voluntary Worker
Ring person no.	1	2	3	4	5	6	7

(a) How often does (PERSON) come?

Show card 19

	CPN	OT	SW	Psychiatrist	Home help	Voluntary Worker	Second Voluntary Worker
4 or more times a week	1	1	1	1	1	1	1
2 or 3 times a week	2	2	2	2	2	2	2
Once a week	3	3	3	3	3	3	3
Less often than once a week but at least once a month	4	4	4	4	4	4	4
Less often than once a month	5	5	5	5	5	5	5

(b) How satisfied or dissatisfied are you with the help or support (PERSON) gives you? Are you

Running prompt

	CPN	OT	SW	Psychiatrist	Home help	Voluntary Worker	Second Voluntary Worker
very satisfied	1	1	1	1	1	1	1
fairly satisfied	2	2	2	2	2	2	2
fairly dissatisfied	3	3	3	3	3	3	3
or very dissatisfied?	4	4	4	4	4	4	4

(c) Ask for voluntary worker(s) if applicable

Which voluntary organisation does (PERSON) come from?

Voluntary worker does not come from any organisation 1

MIND 2

Manic Depression Fellowship 3

Phobic Action/Society 4

National Schizophrenia Fellowship 5

Cruse 6

Alcohol concern 7

Standing conference on Drug Abuse 8

Other 9

18

19

O - N1364B Ma/94 V9

C8 (Can I check), do you have a key worker?

Yes .... 1 → (a)
No 2
Dk .... 3 → (c)

(a) Who is this? [Show card 20]

Social worker 1
Community Psychiatric Nurse (CPN) 2
Occupational Therapist (OT) 3
Psychologist 4
Psychiatrist 5
GP 6
other 7

(b) How often do you see the key worker?

Prompt as necessary

At least once a week 1
Once a fortnight 2
Once a month 3
Once every couple of months 4
Once or twice a year 5
Less than once a year or not at all 6

(c) (Can I check), do you have a care manager?

Yes 1
No 2
Dk 3

Note: Care manager may also be the key worker

C9 [Show card 21]

In the past year, have you been offered any help or support from any of the people listed on this card, or indeed any other service, **which you turned down**?

Yes .... 1 → (a)
No .... 2 → C10

(a) What sort of help/service were you offered?

Code all that apply

Community Psychiatric Nurse 1
Occupational Therapist/Industrial Therapist 2
Social Worker/Counselling Service 3
Psychiatrist 4
Home care worker/Home help 5
Voluntary Worker 6
Key worker/Care manager 7
Other 8

(b) Did you turn it down because you did not want or need the help or for some other reason?

Code all that apply

Did not want/need help 1
Could not face it/handle it 2
Did not like people/not the right people offering help 3
Didn't think it could/would help 4
Inconvenient time or location of service 5
Did not fit in with housing circumstances 6
Other reason 7

20

21

Blank page

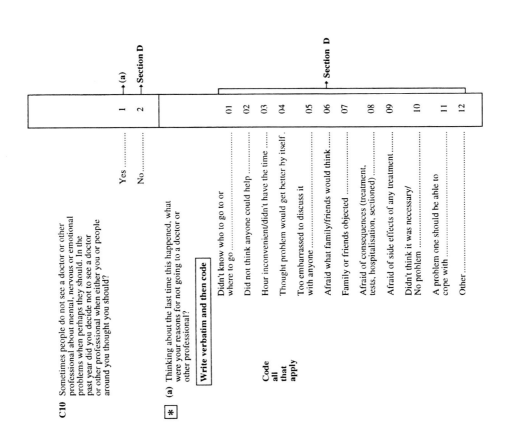

C10 Sometimes people do not see a doctor or other professional about mental, nervous or emotional problems when perhaps they should. In the past year did you decide not to see a doctor or other professional when either you or people around you thought you should?

Yes .... 1 → (a)

No .... 2 → **Section D**

✱ **(a)** Thinking about the last time this happened, what were your reasons for not going to a doctor or other professional?

| Write verbatim and then code |

Code all that apply

Didn't know who to go to or where to go 01

Did not think anyone could help 02

Hour inconvenient/didn't have the time 03

Thought problem would get better by itself 04

Too embarrassed to discuss it with anyone 05

Afraid what family/friends would think .... 06 → **Section D**

Family or friends objected 07

Afraid of consequences (treatment, tests, hospitalisation, sectioned) 08

Afraid of side effects of any treatment 09

Didn't think it was necessary/ No problem 10

A problem one should be able to cope with 11

Other 12

212

22

23

O - N1364B Ma/94 V9

O - N1364B Ma/94 V9

Recent Life Events   DNA: Proxy interviews.... [1] → Go to Section E

The following questions are about events or problems which may have happened to you during the past 6 months which might have caused you distress and to seek help

Use card 22 if subject not alone, otherwise, ask D8 to D13

Then ask (a) if coded 1 at main

	Yes	No	(a) When did this happen? More than 6 months = 6, Less than 1 month = 0. No of months since event
D8 In the past 6 months, have you yourself suffered from a serious illness, injury or an assault?	1	2	☐
D9 (In the past 6 months,) has a serious illness, injury or an assault happened to a close relative?	1	2	☐
D10 (In the past 6 months,) has a parent, spouse (or partner), child, brother or sister of yours died?	1	2	☐
D11 (In the past 6 months,) has a close family friend or another relative died, such as an aunt, cousin or grandparent?	1	2	☐
D12 (In the past 6 months,) have you had a separation due to marital difficulties or broken off a steady relationship?	1	2	☐
D13 (In the past 6 months,) have you had a serious problem with a close friend, neighbour or relative?	1	2	☐

24

Now I'd like to ask you about some other events or problems which may have happened to you during the past 6 months.

Use card 23 if subject not alone, otherwise, ask D14 to D19

Then ask (a) if coded 1 at main

	Yes	No	(a) When did this happen? More than 6 months = 6, Less than 1 month = 0. No of months since event
D14 In the past 6 months, were you made redundant or sacked from your job?	1	2	☐
D15 (In the past 6 months,) were you seeking work without success for more than one month?	1	2	☐
D16 (In the past 6 months,) did you have a major financial crisis, such as losing the equivalent of 3 months income?	1	2	☐
D17 (In the past 6 months,) did you have problems with the police involving a court appearance?	1	2	☐
D18 (In the past 6 months,) was something you valued lost or stolen?	1	2	☐
D19 (Can I check) (In the past 6 months,) did you have to move home and find new accommodation?	1	2	☐

25

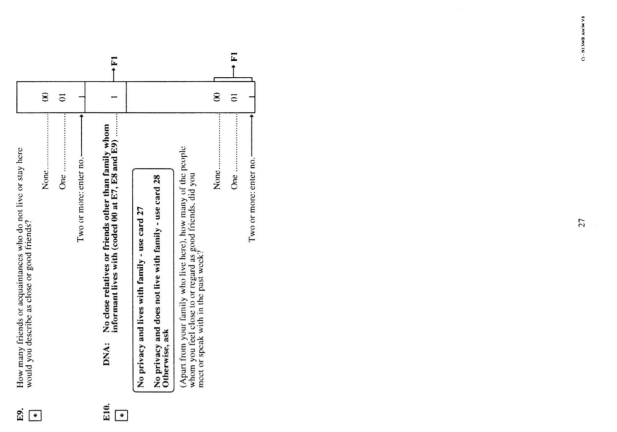

E9. How many friends or acquaintances who do not live or stay here would you describe as close or good friends?

None...... 00
One...... 01
Two or more: enter no. —
→ F1

E10. DNA: No close relatives or friends other than family whom informant lives with (coded 00 at E7, E8 and E9)

No privacy and lives with family - use card 27
No privacy and does not live with family - use card 28
Otherwise, ask

(Apart from your family who live here), how many of the people whom you feel close to or regard as good friends, did you meet or speak with in the past week?

None...... 00
One...... 01
Two or more: enter no. —
→ F1

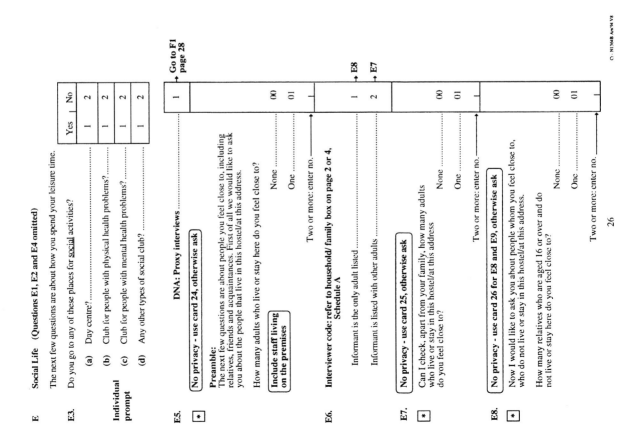

E Social Life (Questions E1, E2 and E4 omitted)

The next few questions are about how you spend your leisure time.

E3. Do you go to any of these places for social activities?

	Yes	No
(a) Day centre?	1	2
(b) Club for people with physical health problems?	1	2
(c) Club for people with mental health problems?	1	2
(d) Any other types of social club?	1	2

Individual prompt

E5. DNA: Proxy interviews ...... 1 → Go to F1 page 28

No privacy - use card 24, otherwise ask

Preamble:
The next few questions are about people you feel close to, including relatives, friends and acquaintances. First of all we would like to ask you about the people that live in this hostel/at this address.

How many adults who live or stay here do you feel close to?

None...... 00
One...... 01
Two or more: enter no. —

Include staff living on the premises

E6. Interviewer code: refer to household/ family box on page 2 or 4, Schedule A

Informant is the only adult listed ...... 1 → E8
Informant is listed with other adults ...... 2 → E7

E7. No privacy - use card 25, otherwise ask

Can I check, apart from your family, how many adults who live or stay in this hostel/at this address do you feel close to?

None...... 00
One...... 01
Two or more: enter no. —

E8. No privacy - use card 26 for E8 and E9, otherwise ask

Now I would like to ask you about people whom you feel close to, who do not live or stay in this hostel/at this address.

How many relatives who are aged 16 or over and do not live or stay here do you feel close to?

None...... 00
One...... 01
Two or more: enter no. —

F   **Education and Employment Status**

F1. At what age did you finish your continuous full-time education at school or college?

Not yet finished	1
Never went to school	2
14 or under	3
15	4
16	5
17	6
18	7
19 or over	8

F2. Please look at this card and tell me whether you have passed any of the qualifications listed. Look down the list and tell me the first one you come to that you have passed.

Show card 29

Degree (or degree level qualification)	1
Teaching qualification	
HNC/HND, BEC/TEC Higher, BTEC Higher	
City and Guilds Full Technological Certificate	2
Nursing qualifications (SRN, SCM, RGN, RM RHV, Midwife)	
'A' levels/SCE higher	
ONC/OND/BEC/TEC **not** higher	
City and Guilds Advanced/Final level	3
'O' level passes (Grade A - C if after 1975)	
GCSE (Grades A - C)	
CSE Grade 1	
SCE Ordinary (Bands A - C)	
Standard Grade (Level 1 - 3)	
SLC Lower	4
SUPE Lower or Ordinary	
School Certificate or Matric.	
City and Guilds Craft/Ordinary level	
CSE Grades 2 - 5	
GCE 'O' level (Grades D & E if after 1975)	
GCSE (Grades D, E, F, G)	
SCE Ordinary (Bands D & E)	5
Standard Grade (Level 4, 5)	
Clerical or commercial qualifications	
Apprenticeship	
CSE ungraded	6
Other qualifications (**specify**)	7
No qualifications	8

Code first that applies

28

29

215

Employment status

F3. Did you do any paid work in the last week, that is in the 7 days ending last Sunday, either as an employee or self employed?

Yes ... 01 → **F5**

No ... → **(a)**

> **Include paid sheltered employment**
> **Include work based training schemes**
> **Exclude college based training schemes**

(a) Even though you weren't working, did you have a job that you were away from last week?

Yes ... 02 → **F4**

No ... → **(i)**

(i) Last week were you:

Code first that applies

waiting to take up a job that you had already obtained? ... 03

looking for work? ... 04

intending to look for work but prevented by **temporary** ill-health, sickness or injury? ... 05

going to school or college full time? **(use only for persons aged 16 - 49)** ... 06

permanently unable to work because of long term sickness or disability? **(for women, use only if aged 16 - 59)** ... 07

retired? **(use only if stopped work at age 50 or over)** ... 08

looking after the home or family? ... 09

or were you doing something else? ... 10

→ **F5**

F4. What was the **main** reason you were away from work (last week)?

Code one only

On leave/holiday ... 1

A mental, nervous or emotional problem ... 2

A physical health problem ... 3

Attending a training course away from the workplace ... 4

Laid off/short time ... 5

Personal/family reason ... 6

Problems with housing ... 7

Other reasons ... 8

→ **F5**

F5. **Interviewer check**

Had a job last week (coded 01 at F3 or 02 at F3(a)) ... 1 → **F8**

Unemployed waiting to take up a job (coded 03 at F3(a)(i)) ... 2 → **F6**

Unemployed looking for work (coded 04 or 05 at F3(a)(i)) ... 3 → **F7**

Others - economically inactive (coded 06 to 10 at F3(a)(i)) ... 4 → **F7**

F6. **Unemployed waiting to take up a job**

Apart from the job you are waiting to take up, have you ever had a paid job or done any paid work?

Yes ... 1 → **F8**

No ... 2 → **See F20, page 36**

F7. **All others unemployed and economically inactive**

(May I check) have you ever had a paid job or done any paid work?

Yes ... 1 → **F8**

No ... 2 → **See F20, page 36**

30   31

216

F11. To those with a job last week (coded 1 at F5, page 31)

DNA: Unemployed/Economically Inactive ...... 1 → See F18, page 36

A. For employees (main job/government scheme)
How long have you been with your present employer (up to yesterday)?

B. For self-employed (main job)
How long have you been self-employed (up to yesterday)?

Show Card 29(b) and prompt as necessary

Less than 4 weeks	01
4 weeks but less than 3 months	02
3 months but less than 6 months	03
6 months but less than 12 months	04
12 months but less than 2 years	05
2 years but less than 3 years	06
3 years but less than 5 years	07
5 years but less than 10 years	08
10 years but less than 15 years	09
15 years but less than 20 years	10
20 years but less than 25 years	11
25 years but less than 30 years	12
30 years but less than 35 years	13
35 years but less than 40 years	14
40 years or more	15

F12. A. For employees (main job/government scheme)

(Introduce if on short time/lay-off:
I'd like to ask about your hours when you are not on short time/laid off ...)

How many hours a week do you usually work (in your main job/government scheme), that is **excluding** meal breaks and overtime?

Check with informant that this is excluding any paid or unpaid overtime → NO OF HOURS excluding meal breaks and overtime

B. For self-employed, (main job)

(Introduce if on short time/lay-off:
I'd like to ask about your hours when you are not on short time/laid off ...)

How many hours a week in total do you usually work (in your main job), that is **excluding** meal breaks but **including** any overtime

Check with informant that this is total hours including any paid or unpaid overtime → TOTAL HOURS excluding meal breaks

If work pattern not based on a week, give average over a few months

33

F8. If employed
(i) What was your job last week?

If not employed
(ii) What was your most recent job?
(iii) What is the job you are waiting to take up?

If retired
(iv) What was your main job?

Job title:

Description:

Industry:

SOC

IND

(a) Informant's Definition

Full-time	1
Part-time	2

(b)

Employee	1	→ F9
Self-employed	2	→ F10

F9 (a) If employee ask or record

Manager	1
Foreman/supervisor	2
other employee	3

(b) How many employees work(ed) in the establishment

1 - 24	1	
25 - 499	2	→ F11
500 or more	3	

F10 If self employed
Do/did you employ other people?

Yes, PROBE:	1 - 24	1
	25 - 499	2
	500 or more	3
No employees		4

32

217

F13. DNA: **Proxy interview** .... 1 → **See F18, page 36**

Earlier I was asking you about how you had been feeling in the past month.

Has your health or the way you have been feeling caused you to take time off work in **the past year**?

Yes .... 1 → **(a)**
No .... 2 → **F14**

(a) How many days in the past year have you taken off work?

Enter number of days ——→

> **Weekends falling within a period of sickness must be included**

F14. **To those with a job last week but temporarily not working because of a mental or physical health problem (coded 2 or 3 at F4, page 30)**

DNA: **Currently working** .... 1 → **Section G, page 38**

How long have you been off work?

Less than 2 weeks 1
2 weeks, less than 1 month 2
1 month, less than 3 months 3
3 months, less than 6 months 4
6 months or more 5

F15. If employee   DNA: **Self-employed (coded 2 at F8(b) page 32)** .... 4 → **F16**

Do you expect to return to your present employer?

Yes .... 1 → **(a)**
No 2
Not sure .... 3 → **F16**

(a) Do you expect to return to the same job?

Yes .... 1 → **Section G, page 38**
No 2
DK 3

F16. Do you expect to be fit to work again?

Yes .... 1 → **F17**
No .... 2 → **Section G, page 38**
Not sure 3

F17. Will you look for another paid job in the future?

Yes .... 1 → **Section G, page 38**
No .... 2 → **(a)**
DK 3

(a) Why will/may you not look for another job?

Code all that apply

No suitable jobs: general employment situation 1
No suitable jobs: due to health problems 2
Too old 3
Housing circumstances make it difficult/impossible 4
Other (**specify**) 5
→ **Section G, page 38**

F20. continued

[*] **(a)** May I just check, would you be able to do some kind of sheltered or part-time work if it were available, or is this impossible?

Could do sheltered work	1	→ **F21**
Could do part-time work	2	→ **F21**
Impossible to do work	3	→ **Section G**

F21. (May I just check) Are you looking for a job at the moment?

Yes	1	→ **F23**
No	2	→ **(a)**

(a) Have you looked for a job at all (since you last worked)?

Yes	1	→ **F22**
No	2	→ **(i)**

[*] **(i)** Why have you not looked for a job?

Code all that apply

No suitable jobs around - general employment situation	1
No suitable jobs for someone with subject's health problem	2
Housing circumstances make it difficult/impossible to get a job	3
Other (specify)	4

→ **Section G**

F22. Why have you stopped looking for jobs?

[*] Code all that apply

No suitable jobs around - general employment situation	1
No suitable jobs for someone with subject's health problem	2
Housing circumstances make it difficult/impossible to get a job	3
Other (specify)	4

F23. Have you ever/since you last worked done any of the following to help get a job:

	Yes	No
Visited a local Job Centre?	1	2
Talked to a Careers Officer?	1	2
Talked to a Disablement Resettlement Officer (DRO)?	1	2

F24 and F25 omitted

F18. **If not working but has worked**

DNA: Never worked (coded 2 at F6 or F7, page 31)	1	→ **See F20**

How old were you when you left your last paid job?

Enter age ──→ **Section G, page 38**

F19.

DNA: Proxy interview	1	→ **Section G, page 38**

[*] Did a mental, nervous or emotional problem have anything to do with your leaving your last job?

Yes	1	→ **(a)**
No	2	→ **See F20**

(a) DNA: Self-employed in last job (coded 2 at F8 (b) page 32) .... 1 → **See F20**

Did your employer ask you to leave or did you leave of your own accord?

Employer asked	1	
Left of own accord	2	→ **See F20**

F20.

DNA: Proxy interview	1	→ **Section G, page 38**
DNA: Retired (code 08 at F3(a)(i), page 30)	2	
DNA: Waiting to take up a job (code 2 at F5, page 31)	3	→ **Section G, page 38**

If not working but not retired

[*] Is the reason that you are not working at present that …

Code first that applies

the way you have been feeling makes it impossible for you to do any kind of paid work?	1	→ **(a)**
a physical health problem makes it impossible for you to do any kind of paid work?	2	→ **F21**
your current housing circumstances make it impossible for you to keep a paid job?	3	
you have not found a suitable paid job?	4	
or because you do not want or need a paid job?	5	→ **Section G, page 38**
Other	6	→ **F21**

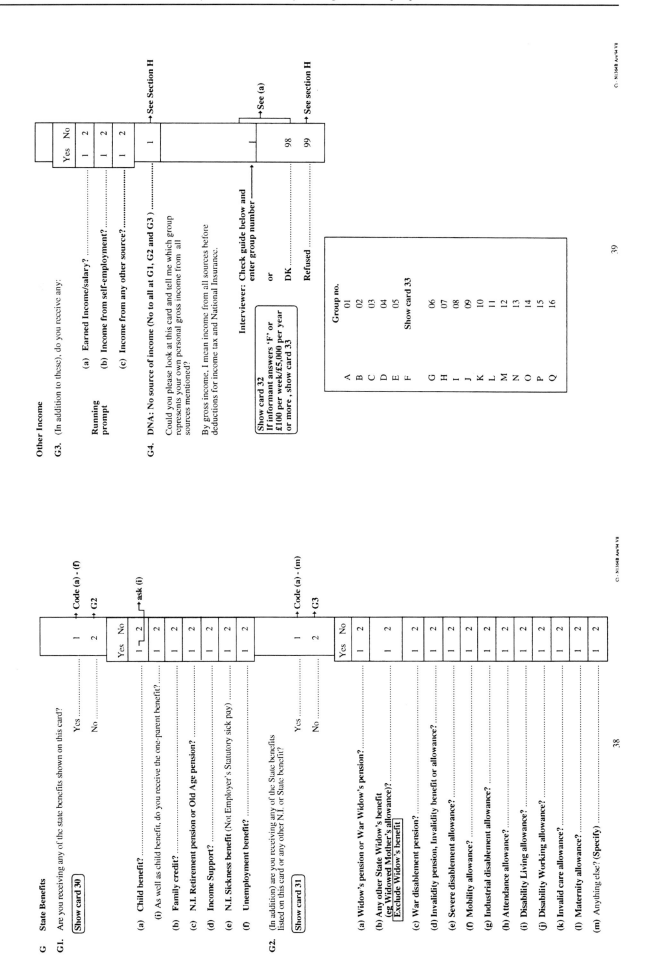

Other Income

G3. (In addition to these), do you receive any:

	Yes	No	
(a) **Earned Income/salary?**	1	2	
(b) **Income from self-employment?**	1	2	
(c) **Income from any other source?**	1	2	→ See Section H

G4. DNA: No source of income (No to all at G1, G2 and G3) ... 1

Could you please look at this card and tell me which group represents your own personal gross income from all sources mentioned?

By gross income, I mean income from all sources before deductions for income tax and National Insurance.

Interviewer: Check guide below and enter group number ——→ or ——→ See (a)

| Show card 32 |
| If informant answers 'F' or |
| £100 per week/£5,000 per year |
| or more, show card 33 |

DK ... 98
Refused ... 99 → See section H

	Group no.
A	01
B	02
C	03
D	04
E	05
F	Show card 33
G	06
H	07
I	08
J	09
K	10
L	11
M	12
N	13
O	14
P	15
Q	16

G State Benefits

G1. Are you receiving any of the state benefits shown on this card?

Show card 30

Yes ... 1 → Code (a) - (f)
No ... 2 → G2

	Yes	No	
(a) **Child benefit?**	1	2	
(i) As well as child benefit, do you receive the one-parent benefit?	1	2	→ ask (i)
(b) **Family credit?**	1	2	
(c) **N.I. Retirement pension or Old Age pension?**	1	2	
(d) **Income Support?**	1	2	
(e) **N.I. Sickness benefit** (Not Employer's Statutory sick pay)	1	2	
(f) **Unemployment benefit?**	1	2	

G2. (In addition) are you receiving any of the State benefits listed on this card or any other N.I. or State benefit?

Show card 31

Yes ... 1 → Code (a) - (m)
No ... 2 → G3

	Yes	No
(a) **Widow's pension or War Widow's pension?**	1	2
(b) **Any other State Widow's benefit** (eg Widowed Mother's allowance)? [Exclude Widow's benefit]	1	2
(c) **War disablement pension?**	1	2
(d) **Invalidity pension, Invalidity benefit or allowance?**	1	2
(e) **Severe disablement allowance?**	1	2
(f) **Mobility allowance?**	1	2
(g) **Industrial disablement allowance?**	1	2
(h) **Attendance allowance?**	1	2
(i) **Disability Living allowance?**	1	2
(j) **Disability Working allowance?**	1	2
(k) **Invalid care allowance?**	1	2
(l) **Maternity allowance?**	1	2
(m) **Anything else?** (Specify)	1	2

38

39

C - N1364B A/v'94 V8

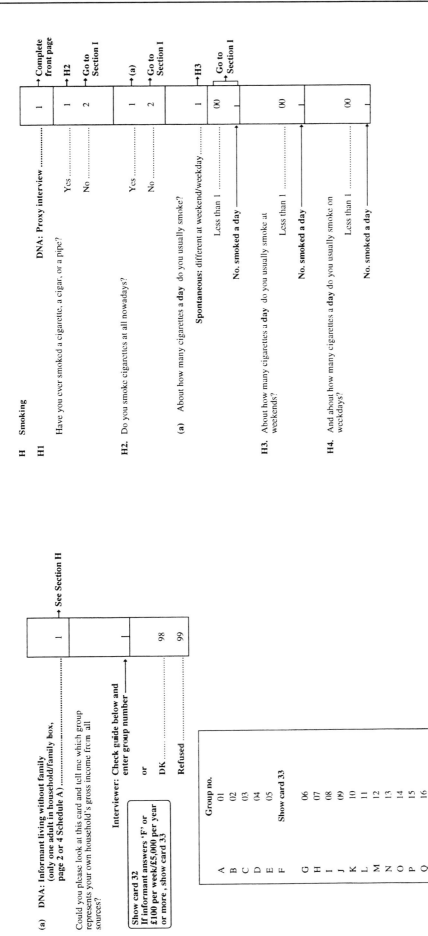

(a) **DNA: Informant living without family**
(only one adult in household/family box,
page 2 or 4 Schedule A) .... → **See Section H**   [1]

Could you please look at this card and tell me which group
represents your own household's gross income from all
sources?

Show card 32
If informant answers 'F' or
£100 per week/£5,000 per year
or more , show card 33

Interviewer: Check guide below and
enter group number ──────→   [ ]

or

DK 98

Refused 99

	Group no.
A	01
B	02
C	03
D	04
E	05
F	Show card 33
G	06
H	07
I	08
J	09
K	10
L	11
M	12
N	13
O	14
P	15
Q	16

O: N1364B Apr'94 V8

H   Smoking

H1
DNA: Proxy interview .... [1] → **Complete**
front page

Have you ever smoked a cigarette, a cigar, or a pipe?
Yes .... [1] → **H2**
No .... [2] → **Go to**
Section I

H2. Do you smoke cigarettes at all nowadays?
Yes .... [1] → **(a)**
No .... [2] → **Go to**
Section I

(a) About how many cigarettes **a day** do you usually smoke?
Spontaneous: different at weekend/weekday .... [1] → **H3**
Less than 1 .... 00 → **Go to**
Section I
No. smoked a day [ ]

H3. About how many cigarettes a **day** do you usually smoke at
weekends?
Less than 1 00
No. smoked a day [ ]

H4. And about how many cigarettes a **day** do you usually smoke on
weekdays?
Less than 1 00
No. smoked a day [ ]

O: N1364B Mar'94 V9

Blank page

222

I   Drinking

11. I'm now going to ask you a few questions about what you drink - that is, if you do drink.

Do you ever drink alcohol nowadays, including drinks you brew or make at home?

Yes	1	→**15**
No	2	→**12**

12. Could I just check, does that mean you never have an alcoholic drink nowadays, or do you have an alcoholic drink very occasionally, perhaps for medicinal purposes or on special occasions like Christmas or New Year?

Very occasionally	1	→**15**
Never	2	→**13**

13. Have you always been a non-drinker, or did you stop drinking for some reason?

Always a non-drinker	1	→**14(a)**
Used to drink but stopped	2	→**14(b)**

14(a).   Always a non drinker

＊ Why is that?

Code all that apply

Religious reasons	1
Don't like it	2
Parent's advice	3
Health reasons	4
Can't afford it	5
Other	6

→ **Go to page 4, Schedule D, then complete front page**

14(b).   Used to drink but stopped

＊ What would you say was the main reason you stopped drinking?

Code all that apply

Religious reasons	1
Don't like it	2
Parent's advice	3
Health reasons	4
Can't afford it	5
Other	6

→ **Go to page 4, Schedule D, then complete front page**

15. I'm going to read out a few descriptions about the amounts of alcohol people drink, and I'd like you to say which one fits you best.
Would you say you:

＊

hardly drink at all	1	
drink a little	2	
drink a moderate amount	3	→**16, page 44**
drink quite a lot	4	
or drink heavily?	5	
DK	6	

42

43

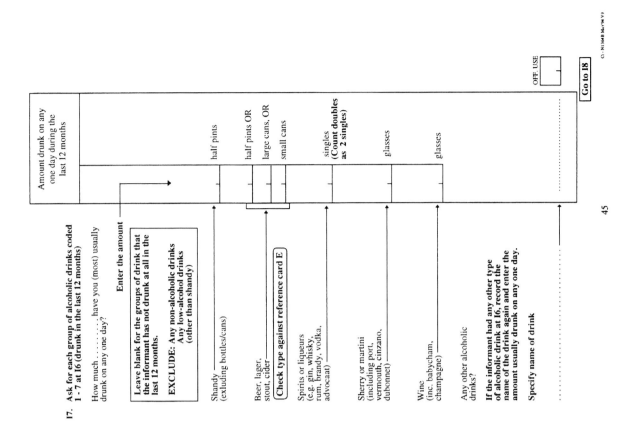

17. Ask for each group of alcoholic drinks coded 1 - 7 at 16 (drunk in the last 12 months)

How much . . . . have you (most) usually drunk on any one day?

Enter the amount

Leave blank for the groups of drink that the informant has not drunk at all in the last 12 months.

EXCLUDE: Any non-alcoholic drinks
Any low-alcohol drinks
(other than shandy)

Drink	Amount drunk on any one day during the last 12 months
Shandy (exluding bottles/cans)	half pints
Beer, lager, stout, cider	half pints OR large cans, OR small cans
Spirits or liqueurs (e.g. gin, whisky, rum, brandy, vodka, advocaat) — Check type against reference card E	singles (Count doubles as 2 singles)
Sherry or martini (including port, vermouth, cinzano, dubonnet)	glasses
Wine (inc. babycham, champagne)	glasses
Any other alcoholic drinks? If the informant had any other type of alcoholic drink at 16, record the name of the drink again and enter the amount usually drunk on any one day. Specify name of drink	

OFF. USE ☐

Go to 18

45

G - N1356B Ma/94 V9

---

16. Show Card 34 and ask for each group of alcoholic drinks listed below:

How often have you had a drink of . . . . . . during the last 12 months?

Ring the appropriate number

EXCLUDE: Any non-alcoholic drinks.
Any low-alcohol drinks
(other than shandy)

Drink	Almost every day	5 or 6 days a week	3 or 4 days a week	Once or twice a week	Once or twice a month	Once every couple of months	Once or twice a year	Not at all in past 12 months
Shandy (exclude bottles/cans)	1	2	3	4	5	6	7	8
Beer, lager, stout, cider	1	2	3	4	5	6	7	8
Spirits or liqueurs (e.g. gin, whisky, rum, brandy, vodka, advocaat)	1	2	3	4	5	6	7	8
Sherry or martini (including port, vermouth, cinzano, dubonnet)	1	2	3	4	5	6	7	8
Wine (inc. babycham, champagne)	1	2	3	4	5	6	7	8
Any other alcoholic drinks? Yes . . . . 1 No . . . . 2 If yes, Specify name of drink	1	2	3	4	5	6	7	8

Go to 17

44

G - N1356B Ma/94 V9

223

I10. During the past year, how often did you have from 5 to 7 **units** of alcoholic drink of any kind in a single day, (that is any combination of beers, glasses of wine, or other alcoholic drinks)?

Show card 34 and use cards 35 and 36 as necessary

Almost every day	1
5 - 6 days a week	2
3 - 4 days a week	3 → Go to Schedule D then complete front page
Once or twice a week	4
Once or twice a month	5
Once every couple of months	6 → Go to page 4, Schedule D then complete front page
Once or twice a year	7
Not at all in the past 12 months	8

47

I8. During the past year, how often did you have 12 or more **units** of alcoholic drink of any kind in a single day, that is any combination of beers, glasses of wine, or other alcoholic drinks?

This card will help you to work out the number of units.

Show card 34 and use cards 35 and 36 as necessary

Almost every day	1
5 - 6 days a week	2
3 - 4 days a week	3 → Go to Schedule D then complete front page
Once or twice a week	4
Once or twice a month	5
Once every couple of months	6
Once or twice a year	7
Not at all in the past 12 months	8 → I9

I9. During the past year, how often did you have from 8 to 11 **units** of alcoholic drink of any kind in a single day, that is any combination of beers, glasses of wine, or other alcoholic drinks?

Show card 34 and use cards 35 and 36 as necessary

Almost every day	1
5 - 6 days a week	2
3 - 4 days a week	3 → Go to Schedule D then complete front page
Once or twice a week	4
Once or twice a month	5
Once every couple of months	6
Once or twice a year	7
Not at all in the past 12 months	8 → I10

46

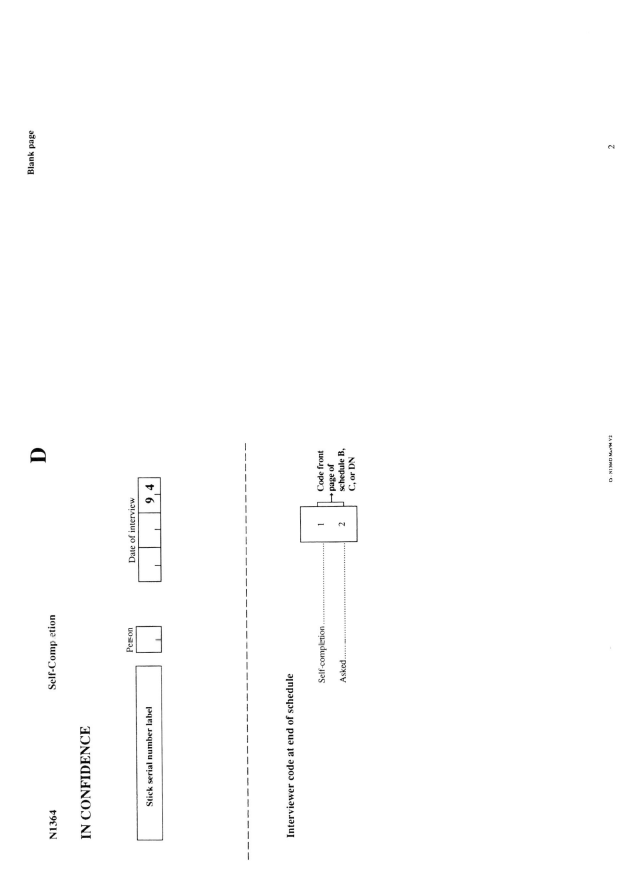

PART A

Here is a list of some experiences that many people have reported in connection with drinking.

Please read each item and indicate if this has ever happened to you in the past 12 months.

> **If you do not drink alcohol at all please go to page 4**

		Please ring 1 or 2 for each item	
		Yes	**No**
1.	I have skipped a number of regular meals while drinking	1	2
2.	I have often had an alcoholic drink the first thing when I got up in the morning	1	2
3.	I have had a strong drink in the morning to get over the effects of the previous night's drinking	1	2
4.	I have woken up the next day not being able to remember some of the things I had done while drinking	1	2
5.	My hands shook a lot after drinking	1	2
6.	I need more alcohol than I used to, to get the same effect as before	1	2
7.	Sometimes I have needed a drink so badly that I couldn't think of anything else	1	2
8.	Sometimes I have woken up during the night or early morning sweating all over because of drinking	1	2
9.	I have stayed drunk for several days at a time	1	2
10.	Once I started drinking it was difficult for me to stop before I became completely drunk	1	2
11.	I sometimes kept on drinking after I promised myself not to	1	2
12.	I deliberately tried to cut down or stop drinking, but I was unable to do so	1	2

3

PART B

Now I'd like to ask about your experience with drugs. Here is a list of the most commonly used drugs.

1. Sleeping Pills, Barbiturates, Sedatives, Downers, Seconal
2. Tranquillisers, Valium, Librium
3. Cannabis, Marijuana, Hash, Dope, Grass, Ganja, Kif
4. Amphetamines, Speed, Uppers, Stimulants, Qat
5. Cocaine, Coke, Crack
6. Heroin, Smack
7. Opiates other than heroin: Demerol, Morphine, Methadone, Darvon, Opium, DF118
8. Psychedelics, Hallucinogens: LSD, Mescaline, Acid, Peyote, Psylocybin (Magic) mushrooms
9. Ecstasy
0. Solvents, inhalants, glue, amyl nitrate

Please look at the above list and answer questions A, B and C

A Have you <u>ever</u> used any of the drugs on the list <u>more than was prescribed for you?</u>

Yes .... 1 → **Go to (i)**
No .... 2 → **Go to question B**

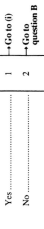

(i) Which of these drugs have you used more than was prescribed for you?
Please circle the category/categories of drugs from the list in the box below.

1	2	3	4	5	6	7	8	9	0

0 → **Go to question B**

Now please answer question B on the opposite page.

4

1. Sleeping Pills, Barbiturates, Sedatives, Downers, Seconal

2. Tranquillisers, Valium, Librium

3. Cannabis, Marijuana, Hash, Dope, Grass, Ganja, Kif

4. Amphetamines, Speed, Uppers, Stimulants, Qat

5. Cocaine, Coke, Crack

6. Heroin, Smack

7. Opiates other than heroin: Demerol, Morphine, Methadone, Darvon, Opium, DF118

8. Psychedelics, Hallucinogens: LSD, Mescaline, Acid, Peyote, Psylocybin (Magic) mushrooms

9. Ecstasy

0. Solvents, inhalants, glue, amyl nitrate

Please answer the following questions thinking about the drugs on this list which you have used without a prescription, to get high, or more than was prescribed for you.

1. Have you ever used any of these drugs more than five times in your life?

Yes .... 1 → **Go to (a)**

No .... 2 → **Go to Q4, page 8**

(a) What was it? (What are they?)
Please circle category/categories of drugs from the list.

[1 2 3 4 5 6 7 8 9 0] → **Go to (b)**

(b) In what year did you first use any of the drugs on this list?

Please enter year → **19** [_ _] → **Go to 2**

B Have you ever used any of the drugs on the list to get high?

Yes .... 1 → **Go to (i)**

No .... 2 → **Go to question C**

(i) Which of these drugs have you used to get high?
Please circle the category/categories of drugs from the list in the box below.

[1 2 3 4 5 6 7 8 9 0] → **Go to question C**

C Have you ever used any of the drugs on the list without a prescription?

Yes .... 1 → **Go to (i)**

No .... 2 → **Go to D**

(i) Which of these drugs have you used without a prescription?
Please circle the category/categories of drugs from the list in the box below.

[1 2 3 4 5 6 7 8 9 0] → **Go to D**

D If you have answered 'yes' to any of questions A, B or C, please go to question 1 on the next page.

If you have answered 'no' to all of questions A, B and C, please hand this back to the interviewer.

2. Have you used any one of these drugs in the past 12 months?

Yes .... 1 → Go to (a)

No .... 2 → Go to Q4, page 8

(a) What was it? (What were they?)
Please circle category/categories of drugs from the list.

| 1 | 2 | 3 | 4 | 5 | 6 | 7 | 8 | 9 | 0 | → Go to Q3 |

3. Have you ever used any one of these drugs every day for two weeks or more in the past 12 months?

Yes .... 1 → Go to (a)

No .... 2 → Go to Q4

(a) What was it? (What were they?)
Please circle category/categories of drugs from the list.

| 1 | 2 | 3 | 4 | 5 | 6 | 7 | 8 | 9 | 0 | → Go to Q4 |

4. May I just check, have you ever injected yourself with drugs?

Yes .... 1 → Go to (a)

No .... 2 → **Thank you for filling this in. Please hand it back to the interviewer.**

(a) Have you ever shared injection equipment with someone else?

Yes .... 1 → Go to Q5

No 2

5. Have you injected a drug in the past month?

Yes .... 1 → Go to (a)

No .... 2 → **Thank you for filling this in. Please hand it back to the interviewer.**

(a) Have you shared injection equipment with someone else in the past month?

Yes 1

No 2

Thank you for filling this in.   Please hand it back to the interviewer.

OPCS, St Catherines House, 10 Kingsway, London WC2B 6JP

O - N1364D May94 V2

O - N1364D May94 V2

N1364 **General Health Self-Completion** **GH**

IN CONFIDENCE

Person [ ] Date of interview [ ] [ ] | [ ] **9 4**

Stick serial number label

Interviewer code at end of schedule

Self-completion 1
Asked 2

Go to question P1, page 11 of A, or page 9 of DN

G:1364GH May94 V5

1

GENERAL HEALTH OVER THE LAST FEW WEEKS

Please read this carefully:

We should like to know how your health has been in general, **over the past few weeks**. Please answer ALL the questions by putting a tick (✓) in the box containing the answer which you think most applies to you.

HAVE YOU RECENTLY ...

GH1 ... been able to concentrate on whatever you're doing?

Better than usual	Same as usual	Less than usual	Much less than usual
1	2	3	4

GH2 ... lost much sleep over worry?

Not at all	No more than usual	Rather more than usual	Much more than usual
1	2	3	4

GH3 ... felt that you are playing a useful part in things?

More so than usual	Same as usual	Less useful than usual	Much less useful
1	2	3	4

GH4 ... felt capable of making decisions about things?

More so than usual	Same as usual	Less so than usual	Much less capable
1	2	3	4

GH5 ... felt constantly under strain?

Not at all	No more than usual	Rather more than usual	Much more than usual
1	2	3	4

GH6 ... felt you couldn't overcome your difficulties?

Not at all	No more than usual	Rather more than usual	Much more than usual
1	2	3	4

G:1364GH May94 V5

2

HAVE YOU RECENTLY . . .

		More so than usual	Same as usual	Less so than usual	Much less than usual
GH7	. . . been able to enjoy your normal day-to-day activities?	[1]	[2]	[3]	[4]

		More so than usual	Same as usual	Less able than usual	Much less able
GH8	. . . been able to face up to your problems?	[1]	[2]	[3]	[4]

		Not at all	No more than usual	Rather more than usual	Much more than usual
GH9	. . . been feeling unhappy and depressed?	[1]	[2]	[3]	[4]

		Not at all	No more than usual	Rather more than usual	Much more than usual
GH10	. . . been losing confidence in yourself?	[1]	[2]	[3]	[4]

		Not at all	No more than usual	Rather more than usual	Much more than usual
GH11	. . . been thinking of yourself as a worthless person?	[1]	[2]	[3]	[4]

		More so than usual	About same as usual	Less so than usual	Much less than usual
GH12	. . . been feeling reasonably happy, all things considered?	[1]	[2]	[3]	[4]

Thank you for filling this in. Now please hand it back to the interviewer.

OPCS, St Catherines House, 10 Kingsway, London, WC2B 6JP

4. What type of hostel is this? Is it a:

Short stay hostel?
Accommodation for homeless people for a few weeks or months. Will accept people with no money; although they may need to be eligible for benefits or wages 1

Low support hostel?
Hostel for people in housing need, but providing only limited support. In many cases staffed only by resident wardens with some catering or maintenance support. Many of these schemes are quite large with a high proportion of single rooms 2

Semi-supportive hostel?
Accommodation for people living fairly independently with some practical or personal support available. There is daytime but not usually 24 hour staff. Emphasis is on finding permanent housing and practical preparation for independent living 3

Supportive hostel?
Accommodation for between 6 - 9 months and a few years. There is a strong emphasis on counselling, education and training to prepare for independent living, and 24 hour staff cover 4

Housing scheme?
Organisation running a number of flats, bedsits or shared houses and offering little more support than sensitive management, for example, helping to organise benefits claims. There is a good chance of permanent housing 5

Supportive Group House?
House offering a community atmosphere and other support services. Great importance is placed on finding the right people for the right houses through a long assessment process 6

Traditional hostel?
Large hostel established for many years and traditionally been used by people who have been homeless for some time. May have dormitory or cubicle accommodation but very few single rooms 7

Or is it some other type of hostel? (Specify) 8

5. Does this establishment cater for:

Single people:

	men and women	1
Code all	men only	2
that apply	women only	3
Prompt as necessary	Families	4

SE - N1364 11s94 V3

2

N1364   **Establishment Schedule**
(Hostels, daycentres, nightshelters)

IN CONFIDENCE

I

Date of Interview

	9	4

Stick serial number label

- -

Interviewer: start at 2. Code 1 at end of sampling

1. Interviewer code at end of sampling

  (i) Transcribe number of eligible residents/visitors from sampling sheet (R or S) →

    Off. use

  (ii) Write sampling interval below (from contact sheet).

    in

    Off. use

    Sampling interval: ....

  (iii) Transcribe number of residents/visitors selected for interview from sampling sheet.(Enter maximum Person number from R, or from column (e) of S) →

2. Interviewer code from observation:

urban	1
rural	2
semi-rural	3

3. Interviewer code:

Nightshelter	1
Daycentre	2
Hostel	3

SE - N1364 11s94 V3

1

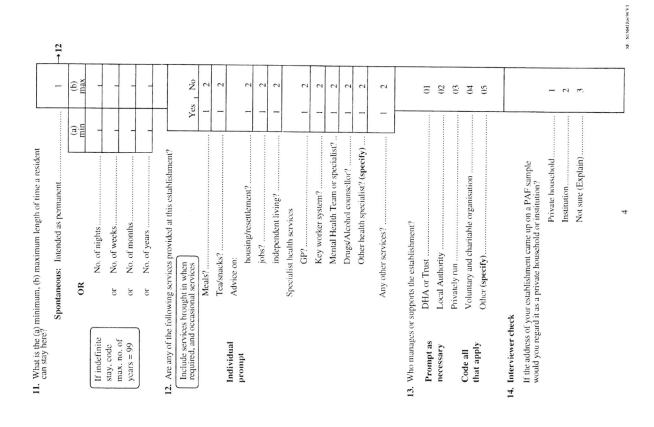

11. What is the (a) minimum, (b) maximum length of time a resident can stay here?

Spontaneous: Intended as permanent ...... 1 → 12

OR

	(a) min	(b) max
No. of nights		
or No. of weeks		
or No. of months		
or No. of years		

If indefinite stay, code max. no. of years = 99

12. Are any of the following services provided at this establishment?

Include services brought in when required, and occasional services

Individual prompt

	Yes	No
Meals?	1	2
Tea/snacks?	1	2
Advice on:		
housing/resettlement?	1	2
jobs?	1	2
independent living?	1	2
Specialist health services		
GP?	1	2
Key worker system?	1	2
Mental Health Team or specialist?	1	2
Drugs/Alcohol counsellor? **(specify)**	1	2
Other health specialist? **(specify)**	1	2
Any other services?	1	2

13. Who manages or supports the establishment?

Prompt as necessary

Code all that apply

DHA or Trust 01
Local Authority 02
Privately run 03
Voluntary and charitable organisation 04
Other (specify) 05

14. Interviewer check

If the address of your establishment came up on a PAF sample would you regard it as a private household or institution?

Private household 1
Institution 2
Not sure (Explain) 3

SF: N13641 Jan '94 V3

4

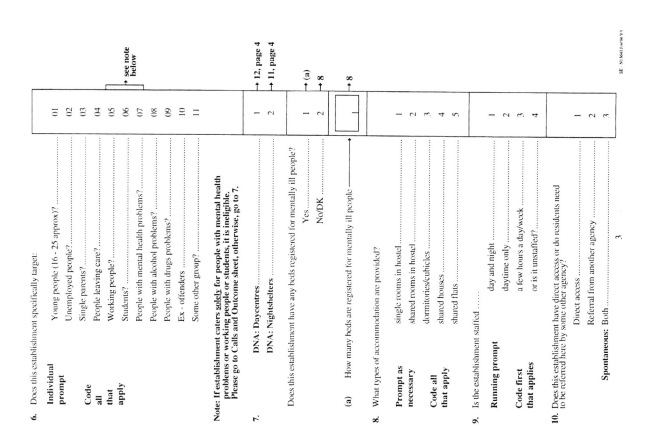

6. Does this establishment specifically target:

Individual prompt

Young people (16 - 25 approx)? 01
Unemployed people? 02
Single parents? 03
People leaving care? 04
Working people? 05
Students? ...... 06 } see note below
People with mental health problems? 07
People with alcohol problems? 08
People with drugs problems? 09
Ex - offenders 10
Some other group? 11

Code all that apply

Note: If establishment caters solely for people with mental health problems or working people or students, it is ineligible. Please go to Calls and Outcome sheet, otherwise, go to 7.

7. DNA: Daycentres ...... 1 → 12, page 4
   DNA: Nightshelters ...... 2 → 11, page 4

Does this establishment have any beds registered for mentally ill people?
Yes ...... 1 → (a)
No/DK ...... 2 → 8

(a) How many beds are registered for mentally ill people → ⬚ → 8

8. What types of accommodation are provided?

Prompt as necessary

single rooms in hostel 1
shared rooms in hostel 2
dormitories/cubicles 3
shared houses 4
shared flats 5

Code all that apply

9. Is the establishment staffed ......

Running prompt

day and night 1
daytime only 2
a few hours a day/week 3
or is it unstaffed? 4

Code first that applies

10. Does this establishment have direct access or do residents need to be referred here by some other agency?

Direct access 1
Referral from another agency 2
Spontaneous: Both 3

SF: N13641 Jan '94 V3

3

Glossary of survey definitions and terms

Adults

In this survey adults were defined as persons aged 16 or over and less than aged 65.

Alcohol consumption

The final classification of alcohol consumption required the amalgamation of detailed information on what alcohol was drunk and the frequency of intake converted into units. The several stages involved in this process were:

1. Establishing how often the subject had the following drinks:

    • **Shandy** (excluding bottles or cans)

    • **Beer, lager, stout or cider**

    • **Spirits or liqueurs** (eg. gin, whisky, rum, brandy, vodka, avocaat)

    • **Wine** (including Babycham and champagne)

    • **Any other alcoholic drink**

2. For any drink taken in the last year, how much was usually drunk on any one day.

3. Converting measures (pints, cans, singles, glasses) into units.

4. Taking account of the different evaluation of units of alcohol for women and men .

The final classification of weekly alcohol consumption was:

    • **Abstainer**

    • **Occasional** - Men (<1); Women (<1)

    • **Light** - Men (1-10); Women (1-7)

    • **Moderate** - Men (11-21); Women (8-14)

• **Fairly heavy** - Men (22-35); Women (15-25)

• **Heavy** - Men (36-50); Women (26-35)

• **Very heavy** - Men (51+); Women (36+)

Alcohol dependence

This was derived from responses to a self-completion questionnaire asked of all survey respondents. Individuals were classified as alcohol dependent if they had three or more positive responses to the following twelve statements. Seven or more positive responses were regarded as indicating severe alcohol dependence.

Loss of control

1. Once I started drinking it was difficult for me to stop before I became completely drunk

2. I sometimes kept on drinking after I had promised myself not to.

3. I deliberately tried to cut down or stop drinking, but I was unable to do so.

4. Sometimes I have needed a drink so badly that I could not think of anything else.

Symptomatic behaviour

5. I have skipped a number of regular meals while drinking

6. I have often had an alcoholic drink the first thing when I got up in the morning.

7. I have had a strong drink in the morning to get over the previous night's drinking

8. I have woken up the next day not being able to remember some of the things I had done while drinking.

9. My hand shook a lot in the morning after drinking.

10. I need more alcohol than I used to get the same effect as before.

11. Sometimes I have woken up during the night or early morning sweating all over because of drinking.

Binge Drinking

12. I have stayed drunk for several days at a time.

Antipsychotic drugs
These are also known as 'neuroleptics'. In the short term they are used to quieten disturbed patients whatever the underlying psychopathology.
See Depot Injections

Cigarette smoking
Questions on cigarette smoking were taken from the General Household Survey. For those who did smoke the average number of cigarettes smoked per day was calculated from answers to questions on the number of cigarettes usually smoked on weekdays and on weekends. The final classification did not take account of the tar level of cigarettes, only the quantity smoked:

• **Light smoker** - less than 10 a day

• **Moderate smoker** - more than 10 but less than 20 a day

• **Heavy smoker** - at least 20 a day

• **Ex-regular smoker**

• **Never a regular smoker**

Depot injections
When antipsychotic medication is given by injections on a monthly basis, these are sometimes termed depot injections.

Drug dependence
This was derived from responses to a self-completion questionnaire asked of all survey respondents. Individuals were classified as drug dependent if they gave a positive response to the question: Have you ever used any one of these drugs every day for two weeks or more in the past 12 months? The list of 10 categories of drug is shown in the box below. A prerequisite was that the drugs must have been taken either without a prescription, more than what was prescribed for the subject, or to get high.

1. Sleeping Pills, Barbiturates, Sedatives, Downers, Seconal
2. Tranquillisers, Valium, Librium
3. Cannabis, Marijuana, Hash, Dope, Grass, Ganja, Kif
4. Amphetamines, Speed, Uppers, Stimulants, Qat
5. Cocaine, Coke, Crack
6. Heroin, Smack
7. Opiates other than heroin: Demerol, Morphine, Methadone, Darvon, Opium, DF118
8. Psychedelics, Hallucinogens: LSD, Mescaline, Acid, Peyote, Psylocybin (Magic) mushrooms
9. Ecstasy
10. Solvents, inhalants, glue, amyl nitrate

Drug use
Information was initially collected on the use of particular groups of drugs. This was subsumed under more general headings for the purpose of analysis.

• **Cannabis**

• **Stimulants** (cocaine and speed)

• **Hallucinogens** (acid and Ecstasy)

• **Hypnotics** (barbiturates, sedatives, tranquillisers, valium, librium, etc)

• **Other** - heroin, opium, solvents

A subject was classified as having used drugs in the past year if he/she had taken any of these drugs in the past 12 months either without a prescription, more than was prescribed, or to get high, and had taken the drug more than five times in his/her life.

Economic activity
The questions used to measure economic activity were taken from those regularly asked in the General Household Survey. All adults are placed into one of eight categories:

- **Working** - having done paid work in the seven days ending the Sunday before the interview, either as an employee or self-employed, including those were not actually at work but had a job they were away from.

- **Looking for work**

- **Intending to look for work** but prevented by temporary, ill-health, sickness or injury

- **Going to school or college full-time** - only used for persons aged 16-49.

- **Permanently unable to work** due to long-term sickness or disability - for women, only used if aged 16-59

- **Retired** - used only if stopped work at the aged of 50 or over

- **Looking after the home or family**

- **Other** - doing something else

Educational level
Educational level was based on the highest educational qualification obtained and was grouped as follows:

Degree (or degree level qualification)

Teaching, HND, Nursing
Teaching qualification
HNC/HND, BEC/TEC Higher, BTEC Higher
City and Guilds Full Technological Certificate

Nursing qualifications:
(SRN,SCM,RGN,RM,RHV, Midwife)

A level
GCE A-levels/SCE higher
ONC/OND/BEC/TEC/not higher
City and Guilds Advanced/Final level
O level
GCE O-level (grades A-C if after 1975)
GCSE (grades A-C)
CSE (grade 1)
SCE Ordinary (bands A-C)
Standard grade (levels 1-3)
SLC Lower SUPE Lower or Ordinary
School certificate or Matric
City and Guilds Craft/Ordinary level

GCSE/CSE
GCE O-level (grades D-E if after 1975)
GCSE (grades D-G)
CSE (grades 2-5)
SCE Ordinary (bands D-E)
Standard grade (levels 4-5)
Clerical or commercial qualifications
Apprenticeship
Other qualifications

No qualifications
CSE ungraded
No qualifications

Employment status
Four types of employment status were identified: working full time, working part time, unemployed and economically inactive.

Working adults
The two categories of working adults include persons who did any work for pay or profit in the week ending the last Sunday prior to interview, even if it was for as little as one hour, including Saturday jobs and casual work (e.g. babysitting, running a mail order club).

Self-employed persons were considered to be working if they worked in their own business for the purpose of making a profit, or even if the enterprise was failing to make a profit or just being set up.

235

Anyone on a Government scheme which was employer based was also 'working last week'.

Informants' definitions dictated whether they felt they were working full time or part time.

Unemployed adults
This category included those who were waiting to take up a job that had already been obtained, those who were looking for work, and people who intended to look for work but were prevented by temporary ill-health, sickness or injury. 'Temporary' was defined by the informant.

Economically inactive
This category comprised five main categories of people:

Going to school or college' only applied to people who were under 50 years of age. The category included people following full-time educational courses at school or at further education establishments (colleges, university, etc). It included all school children (16 years and over).

During vacations, students were treated as 'going to school or college' even where their return to college was dependent on passing a set of exams. If however, they were having a break from full-time education, i.e. they were taking a year out, they were not counted as being in full-time education.

Permanently unable to work because of long-term sickness or disability' only applied to those under state retirement age, ie to men aged 16 to 64 and to women aged 16 to 59. 'Permanently' and 'long-term' were defined by the informant.

'Retired' only applied to those who retired from their full-time occupation at age 50 or over and were not seeking further employment of any kind.

'Looking after the home or family' covered anyone who was mainly involved in domestic duties, provided this person had not already been coded in an earlier category.

'Doing something else' included anyone for whom the earlier categories were inappropriate.

Ethnicity
Adults (including household members) were classified into nine groups by the informant.

White	White
Black - Caribbean Black - African Black - Other	West Indian/African
Indian Pakistani Bangladeshi Chinese	Asian/Oriental
None of these	Other

For analysis purpose these nine groups were subsumed under 4 headings: White, West Indian/African, Asian/Oriental and Other.

Family unit
In order to classify the relationships of the subject to other members of the household in hostels and PSLA, the household members were divided into family units.

Subjects were assigned to a family unit depending on whether they were or ever had been married, and whether they (or their partners) had any children living with them.

A 'child' was defined for family unit purposes as an adult who lives with one or two parents, provided he or she has never been married and has no child of his or her own in the household.

For example, a household containing three women: a grandmother, mother and child would contain two family units with the mother and child being in one unit, and the grandmother being in another. Hence family units can consist of:

- A married or cohabiting couple or a lone parent with their children

- Other married or cohabiting couples

- An adult who has previously been married. If the adult is now living with parents, the parents are treated as being in a separate family unit

- An adult who does not live with either a spouse, partner, child or parent. This can include adults who live with siblings or with other unrelated people, e.g. flatmates.

Family unit type
Each informant's family unit was classified into one of six family unit types:

'Couple no children' included a married or cohabiting couple without children.

'Couple with child' comprised a married or cohabiting couple with at least one child from their liaison or any previous relationship.

'Lone parent' describes both men and women (who may be single, widowed, divorced or separated) living with at least one child. The subject in this case could be a divorced man looking after his 12 year-old son or a 55 year-old widow looking after a 35 year-old, daughter who had never married and had no children of her own.

'One person' describes the family unit type and does not necessarily mean living alone. It includes people living alone but includes one person living with a sister, or the grandmother who is living with her daughter and her family. It also includes adults living with unrelated people in shared houses, e.g. flatmates.

'Adult living with parents' describes a family unit which has the same members as 'couple with child' but in this case it is the adult son or daughter who is the subject. It includes a 20 year old unmarried student living with married or cohabiting parents, and a 62 year old single woman caring for her elderly parents.

'Adult living with lone parent' covers the same situations as above except that there is one and not two parents in the household.

Marital status
Informants were categorised according to their own perception of marital status. Married and cohabiting took priority over other categories. Cohabiting included anyone living together with their partner as a couple.

Physical complaints
Informants were asked 'Do you have any long-standing illness, disability or infirmity? By long-standing I mean anything that has troubled you over a period of time or that is likely to affect you over a period of time?'

Those that answered yes to this question were then asked 'What is the matter with you?'; interviewers were asked to try and obtain a medical diagnosis, or to establish the main symptoms. From these responses, illnesses were coded to the site or system of the body that was affected, using a classification system that roughly corresponded to the chapter headings of the International Classification of Diseases (ICD–10). Some of the illnesses identified were mental illnesses and these were excluded from the classification of physical illness. Physical illness did, however, include physical disabilities and sensory complaints such as eyesight and hearing problems.

Primary support group
In hostels and PSLA the size of the individual's primary support group was calculated as a measure of the extent of their social networks. In the survey, data were collated about the size of four groups of people who respondents said they felt close to:

- Adult family members living with the respondent

- Adults who lived with the respondent, including staff living on the premises

- Relatives who did not live with the respondent

- Friends and acquaintances who did not live with the respondent that could not be described as close or good friends

The total number of close friends and relatives

were regarded as the individual's primary support group. For the purposes of analysis, the total number in the primary support group was categorised into: 3 or fewer, 4-8, and 9 or more.

Psychiatric morbidity

The expression psychiatric morbidity refers to the degree or extent of the prevalence of mental health problems within a defined area.

Social class

Based on the Registrar General's 1991 *Standard Occupational Classification,* Volume 3 OPCS, HMSO: London social class was ascribed on the basis of the following priorities:

Social class was based on the informant's own occupation. Secondly, social class was based on the informant's current occupation or, if the informant was unemployed or economically inactive at the time of interview but had previously worked, social class was based on the most recent previous occupation.

The classification used in the tables is as follows:

Descriptive definition	Social class
Professional	I
Intermediate occupations	II
Skilled occupations — non-manual	III NM
Skilled occupations — manual	III M
Partly-skilled	IV
Unskilled occupations	V
Armed Forces	

Social class was not determined where the subject (and spouse) had never worked, or if the subject was a full-time student or where occupation was inadequately described.

Stressful life events

Questions on stressful life events were only asked of residents in hostels and private sector leased accommodation.

Responses of 'yes' to any of the following 11 questions identified a recent stressful life event.

In the past 6 months...

1. have you yourself suffered from a serious illness, injury or an assault?

2. has a serious illness, injury or an assault happened to a close relative?

3. has a parent, spouse (or partner), child, brother or sister of yours died?

4. has a close family friend or another relative died, such as an aunt, cousin or grandparent?

5. have you had a separation due to marital difficulties or broken off a steady relationship?

6. have you had a serious problem with a close friend, neighbour or relative?

7. were you made redundant or sacked from your job?

8. were you seeking work without success for more than one month?

9. did you have a major financial crisis, such as losing the equivalent of 3 months income?

10. did you have problems with the police involving a court appearance?

11. was something you valued lost or stolen?

Informants were classified according to the number of stressful life events they had experienced in the last 6 months.

Informants were also asked:

12. did you have to move home and find new accommodation?

Printed in the United Kingdom for HMSO
Dd302351 4/96 C18 G5600 10170